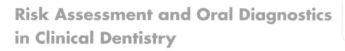

Risk Assessment and Oral Diagnostics in Clinical Dentistry

Risk Assessment and Oral Diagnostics in Clinical Dentistry

Dena J. Fischer
Nathaniel S. Treister
Andres Pinto

WILEY-BLACKWELL

A John Wiley & Sons, Inc., Publication

Editorial Offices

2121 State Avenue, Ames, Iowa 50014-8300, USA

The Atrium, Southern Gate, Chichester, West Sussex, PO19 8SQ, UK

9600 Garsington Road, Oxford, OX4 2DQ, UK

For details of our global editorial offices, for customer services and for information about how to apply for permission to reuse the copyright material in this book please see our website at www.wiley.com/wiley-blackwell.

Library of Congress Cataloging-in-Publication Data

Fischer, Dena Joi.
  Risk assessment and oral diagnostics in clinical dentistry / Dena J. Fischer, Nathaniel S. Treister, Andres Pinto.
    p. ; cm.
  Includes bibliographical references and index.
  ISBN 978-0-8138-2118-4 (pbk. : alk. paper) – ISBN 978-1-118-48324-4 (ePDF/ebook) –
ISBN 978-1-118-48327-5 (ePub) – ISBN 978-1-118-48338-1 (mobi)
I. Treister, Nathaniel S. II. Pinto, Andres, 1972– III. Title.
[DNLM: 1. Diagnosis, Oral–methods. 2. Dentistry–methods. 3. Mouth Diseases–diagnosis.
4. Risk Assessment. WU 141]
617.6′01–dc23

                                   2012029835

A catalogue record for this book is available from the British Library.

Cover image (left): © bojan fatur
Cover design by Nicole Teut

Set in 10/12pt Times by SPi Publisher Services, Pondicherry, India
Printed and bound in Singapore by Markono Print Media Pte Ltd

Disclaimer

1   2013

Contents

Authors

Dena J. Fischer, DDS, MSD, MS
Assistant Professor
University of Illinois at Chicago College
of Dentistry
Department of Oral Medicine and
Diagnostic Sciences
Chicago, Illinois

Nathaniel S. Treister, DMD, DMSC
Assistant Professor of Oral Medicine
Director of Postgraduate Oral Medicine
Harvard School of Dental Medicine
Associate Surgeon
Brigham and Women's Hospital
Boston, Massachusetts

Andres Pinto, DMD, MPH, FDS, RCSED
Associate Professor of Oral Medicine and
Community Health
Director of Oral Medicine Services
University of Pennsylvania, School of
Dental Medicine
Attending Physician
The Children's Hospital of Philadelphia
Hospital of the University of Pennsylvania,
Perelman School of Medicine
Philadelphia, Pennsylvania

Preface

For the past few decades, the United States and world populations have increased, partly because people are living longer, resulting in individuals with chronic disease living long and robust lives. Many medical conditions can have an impact upon oral health and/or the safe delivery of dental care. For example, a patient with diabetes has an increased risk of developing periodontal disease, or a patient with a history of atrial fibrillation on prophylactic anticoagulant medication may be at a greater risk of post-operative bleeding following a surgical procedure. Consequently, oral health care providers need to be comfortable with assessing the risk of providing dental care to their patients with systemic disease as well as evaluation of oral conditions that may represent manifestations or consequences of systemic disease. This clinical guide will address these two major topics. First, we will discuss guidelines for risk assessment of systemic conditions that may complicate or be complicated by dental treatment. Next, we will review guidelines for diagnosis of oral conditions to assist in the diagnosis of orofacial conditions within the scope of dental practice.

Risk assessment of systemic health is of key importance and should be addressed upon first interaction between a dental provider and patient. After obtaining a thorough medical history (chapter 1) and vital signs (chapter 2), patients should be assessed for their potential for bleeding (chapter 3), potential for infection (chapter 4), potential for poor wound healing (chapter 5) and their general ability to withstand dental treatment. Patients with signs and symptoms of suspected disease or known disease that is not well managed require referral to a medical provider for thorough evaluation prior to providing elective dental care.

In patients with known medical conditions, diagnostic testing is typically utilized to monitor disease status and response to or compliance with treatment. In the first section of this clinical guide, we will discuss the common diagnostic tests utilized in medical settings, the interpretation of abnormal test values, and the clinical implications of abnormal findings. Dental providers should have a thorough understanding of and ability to interpret the results of diagnostic tests to better communicate with medical colleagues and to understand the disease status of their patients.

The second section of this clinical guide addresses diagnosis of orofacial disease and oral manifestations of systemic disease. Following a thorough extraoral and intraoral clinical examination, hard and/or soft tissue abnormalities should be assessed through the diagnostic process, which involves determining a differential diagnosis while taking into consideration the disease process and the system/tissue/cell type(s) involved. We will review clinical signs and symptoms of common oral conditions as well as diagnostic tests and procedures that can be utilized to determine a definitive diagnosis. The definitive diagnosis is essential in developing a plan of treatment and time interval for follow-up and monitoring.

We hope this clinical guide will be a useful tool for dental students in training, dental residents, and practicing dentists throughout the span of their professional lives. It has been designed to be an easy-to-use reference with features such as clinical images, alert boxes, and guidelines, so that the busy clinician can quickly look up information about his/her patients to assist in guiding appropriate treatment. While the majority of dental patients can be treated with minimal risk of complications, dentists must be well informed and confident to fully address the oral health care considerations of their entire practice.

Dena J. Fischer, DDS, MSD, MS
Nathaniel S. Treister, DMD, DMSc
Andres Pinto, DMD, MPH, FDS, RCSEd

Acknowledgements

With love and gratitude to our families, colleagues, and most importantly our patients, who provided us with the expertise to develop this clinical guide.

Part A

Guidelines for Risk Assessment of Systemic Conditions that may Complicate or be Complicated by Dental Treatment

1 Basics of the Health History, Physical Examination, and Clinical Investigations

1.0 INTRODUCTION

This chapter sets the foundation for this clinical guide by describing the basic principles and processes of clinical evaluation of the patient. Risk assessment first and foremost depends on obtaining a comprehensive medical history. In addition to physical examination, the clinician must determine whether any other clinical investigations are indicated prior to providing oral health care. These elements provide an essential basis for the clinical guide.

1.1 Obtaining a complete medical history

A wide variety of medical conditions and their treatments have the potential to affect oral health and may require specific considerations prior to providing dental care. In order to adequately assess a patient's health and determine risk for developing complications, a complete medical history must be obtained and updated on a regular basis. Whether paper or electronic medical records are utilized, this information should be clear and easy to locate. Contact information for the patient's primary care physician and any relevant medical specialists should also be recorded and accessible. Details of all telephone, email, or mail correspondences with the patient or his/her medical providers, as well as laboratory reports, should be included in the patient's chart.

   While a self-completed health history form can be useful in screening for certain medical conditions and risks, this should be used to guide, rather than replace, the medical interview. The oral health care provider and patient should be facing each other in a comfortable and relaxed manner during the interview, and translators should be used when necessary. When there are any questions or items in the medical history requiring greater detail or clarification, the patient's primary care physician should be consulted.

1.1.1 Chief complaint

The chief complaint is the patient's primary reason for seeking medical/dental consultation and should be recorded in his/her own words. Sometimes, a patient's chief complaint when he/she presents to his/her oral health care provider will be some type of oral pain or a

Risk Assessment and Oral Diagnostics in Clinical Dentistry, First Edition.
Dena J. Fischer, Nathaniel S. Treister and Andres Pinto.
© 2013 John Wiley & Sons, Inc. Published 2013 by John Wiley & Sons, Inc.

complication of a recent dental procedure. In some cases, the chief complaint may be directly related to an underlying medical condition. Examples include a patient with salivary gland hypofunction and rampant dental caries, or a patient with acute leukemia and acute onset of gingival bleeding.

1.1.2   History of present illness

The history of present illness relates directly to the chief complaint and is told from the perspective of the patient. This is essentially the story describing the chief complaint and should be collected in sufficient detail. Basic elements should include, as relevant to the nature of the chief complaint: history of onset; the duration, nature, quality, and timing of symptoms; complications; pain score; modifying factors; any treatment provided; and whether symptoms are stable, improving, or deteriorating.

1.1.3   Past medical history

The past medical history includes all relevant aspects of a patient's health history both past and present. Medical conditions for which a patient has received treatment, or is actively being treated, and overall continuity of medical care should be included. Pertinent details of treatment and overall management should be obtained, such as timing of chemotherapy cycles in a patient undergoing cancer therapy, hemodialysis schedule in a patient with renal failure, or glycated hemoglobin (HbA1c) levels in a diabetic patient.

1.1.4   Medications and allergies

All current medications, prescription and non-prescription (over-the-counter, herbal supplements), taken on a regular basis must be listed. The dose, schedule, and most recent dose taken should also be noted, in particular if the medication is immunosuppressive/immunomodulatory, antihypertensive, antiglycemic, antithrombotic, or anticoagulatory. Previous exposure to specific medications, such as antiresorptive agents (e.g., bisphosphonates), is also important and should be selectively collected. If there appear to be any inconsistencies between the patient's medical history and the list of medications, clarification should be requested. All reported drug allergies must be clearly noted, including the specific allergic reaction. Expected adverse side effects, such as gastrointestinal upset with opioid analgesics, should not be misclassified as an "allergy," even if reported as such by the patient (adverse drug reactions).

Certain medications have the potential to interact with one another through competitive binding, or through induction or inhibition of the hepatic cytochrome p450 pathway. Some common examples, such as antibiotics, antifungals, and analgesics, are shown in Table 1.1.

1.1.5   Review of systems

The review of systems is an extension of the past medical history that serves more or less as a "checklist" of a patient's overall health by assessing specific symptoms within each system in a comprehensive manner. Systems include neurologic/psychiatric; ears, eyes, nose, and throat (EENT); cardiovascular/respiratory; musculoskeletal; hematologic; endocrine; gastrointestinal; and genitourinary (Table 1.2). Any positive responses should be followed with additional questioning and the patient should be referred to his/her primary care physician for further evaluation when indicated.

Table 1.1 Cytochrome P450-associated drug interactions.

	Substrates	Inhibitors	Inducers
Mechanism	Metabolism CYP450 dependent	May potentiate activity of CYP450 substrates by decreasing metabolism	May reduce efficacy of CYP450 substrates by increasing metabolism
Class of Medication			
Antiasthmatics	Theophylline		
Antibiotics	Clarithromycin, erythromycin	Ciprofloxacin, clarithromycin, erythromycin, ofloxacin, metronidazole	Rifmapin, isoniazid
Anticoagulants	Warfarin		
Anticonvulsants	Phenytoin, carbamazepine		Carbamazepine, phenytoin
Antidepressants	Amitriptyline, desipramine, imipramine, paroxitene	Fluoxetine, fluvoxamine, paroxitene, sertraline	
Antifungals		Clotrimazole, fluconazole, itraconazole, ketoconazole	
Antipsychotics	Halperidol, pimozide, risperidone		
Barbiturates			Phenobarbital, secobarbital
Benzodiazepines	Alprazolam, diazepam, midazolam, triazolam		
Cardiac medications	Amlodipine, diltiazem, felodipine, verapamil, metoprolol, propranolol,timolol	Diltiazem, verapamil	Amiodarone
Corticosteroids	Hydrocortisone, methylprednisolone		Dexamethasone, hydrocortisone, prednisolone, methylprednisolone
Food		Grapefruit juice, Seville oranges	
H2 receptor blockers		Cimetidine	
Herbal medications			St John's wort
HIV medications	Idinavir, nelfinavir, ritonavir, saquinavir	Idinavir, nelfinivir, ritonavir, saquinavir	Efavirenz, nevirapine
Hormones	Estrogens, progestins		
Hypoglycemic agents	Glipizide, glyburide, tolbutamide		Pioglitazone, troglitizone
Immunosuppressive agents	Cyclosporine, tacrolimus		
Narcotic analgesics	Codeine, hydrocodone, tramadol		
Non-narcotic analgesics	Acetaminophen, diclofenac, ibuprofen, naproxen		
Statins	Atorvastatin, lovastatin, simvastatin		

Table 1.2   Potentially serious drug interactions that may interact with medications prescribed by oral health care providers.

Medication	Potential effect	Medications at risk for interaction	Guidelines
Warfarin	Increased INR	Ciprofloxacin, clarithromycin, erythromycin, metronidazole, trimethoprim-sulfamethoxazole	Select alternative antibiotic
		Acetaminophen, acetylsalicylic acid, NSAIDs	Minimize dose, monitor INR, best to avoid NSAIDs entirely
Fluoroqinolones	Decreased absorption of fluoroquinolone	Divalent/trivalent cations or sucralfate	Can safely space administration by 2–4 hours
Carbamazepine	Increased carbamazepine levels	Cimetidine, erythromycin, clarithromycin, fluconazole	Monitor carbamazepine levels
	Decreased carbamazepine levels	Rifampin	
Phenytoin	Increased phenytoin levels	Cimetidine, erythromycin, clarithromycin, fluconazole	Monitor phenytoin levels
	Decreased phenytoin levels	Rifmampin	
Phenobarbital	Increased phenobarbital levels	Cimetidine, erythromycin, clarithromycin, fluconazole	Monitor phenobarbital levels
	Decreased phenobarbital levels	Rifampin	
Lithium	Increased lithium levels	NSAIDs	Consider lowering lithium dose, monitor levels
Oral contraceptives	Decreased efficacy of oral contraceptive	Antibiotics	Use of alternative contraceptive method
Sildenafil	Increased sildenafil levels	Cimetidine, erythromycin, itraconazole, ketoconazole	Dose reduce sildenafil
HMG-CoA reductase inhibitor	Increased risk of rhabdomyolysis	Erythromycin, itraconazole	Avoid combination
SSRIs	Increased risk of seizures, serotonin syndrome	Tramadol	Avoid combination

1.1.6   *Family and social history*

The family history should include any significant known medical conditions in first-degree relatives or that have been present in multiple generations. The social history should include whether the patient is single, previously married and/or divorced, or in a long-term relationship, and if s/he has children, as well as any other pertinent details that might impact his/her overall health. In addition, the patient's occupation is important. For those who are not working, it is important to understand why, as this may be related to an underlying medical condition. Tobacco history should be obtained in pack-years (packs per day times the number of years), and if the patient has discontinued use, for how long; regular use of marijuana should also be ascertained. Alcohol and recreational drug use history should include amount and frequency and whether there is any history of treatment for abuse, addiction, or dependency. These aspects of the social history are important as stress, lifestyle, and psychosocial factors may contribute to disease presentation and may impact management.

1.1.7   Past dental history

A patient's past dental history provides a great deal of information with respect to future risk of developing dental disease and associated complications. This should include whether care has been routine and preventive, or sporadic and problem-driven, and if so, why. Oral hygiene practices, home care, and diet should be reviewed.

1.2   Physical examination

Vital signs, including at minimum blood pressure and pulse, should be collected on all new patients and on an annual basis for general health screening, with appropriate referral when findings are abnormal (see chapter 2). For oral health care providers, the physical examination is largely limited to the head and neck and the oral cavity, intraorally extending from the labial mucosa anteriorly, to the soft palate, tonsils, and visible oropharynx posteriorly. Limited dermatologic examination, for example, can often be informative, especially when there is a chief complaint of oral lesions and concurrent skin lesions. Similarly, a limited neurologic examination may be warranted in a patient with signs and symptoms suggestive of a central nervous system disorder (Figure 1.1; see Figure 9.2). For proper conduct of a comprehensive examination, nothing more is needed than a good light source, a mouth mirror and gauze, which can be useful for manipulating the tongue and assessing salivary gland function. Normal findings should be summarized and for all positive findings, the size must be recorded as well as a description of color, consistency and contours of tissues.

1.2.1   Extraoral examination

Extraoral examination begins with careful visual inspection for skin changes and any head/neck asymmetry or swelling (Figure 1.2). The head and neck is then palpated for swelling, tenderness, lymphadenopathy, thyromegaly, and any other abnormalities. Temporomandibular joint examination includes observation of opening, closing, and lateral excursions of the jaw, palpation of the muscles of mastication, and evaluation of the joints for sounds and tenderness (see chapter 12). Depending on the chief complaint and history of present illness, a limited or more extensive cranial nerve examination may be included to evaluate for neuromuscular and neurosensory deficits.

1.2.2   Intraoral examination

The intraoral soft tissues should be examined thoroughly, including the upper and lower labial mucosa, right and left buccal mucosa, vestibules, gingiva, ventrolateral and dorsal surfaces of the tongue, floor of mouth, hard and soft palate, and the tonsils and oropharynx.

(a)

(b)

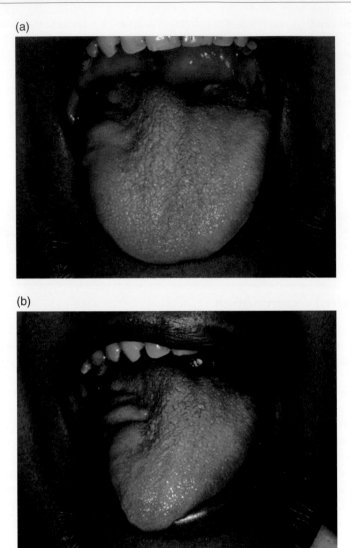

Figure 1.1   62-year-old male with metastatic prostate cancer involving the clivus (affecting cranial nerves IX and XII on the right side) with progressive right-sided tongue and constrictor muscle weakness. Straight protrusion of the tongue (a) demonstrates right-sided muscle flaccidity, whereas excursion to the right side (b) demonstrates minimal movement.

Normally keratinized sites include the gingiva, hard palate, and tongue dorsum; these sites have a thicker, paler appearance than the rest of the non-keratinized mucosa that tends to be more pink or red in color. The mucosa should be assessed for red and/or white changes, pigmentation, ulceration, or any other abnormalities (Figure 1.3). These tissues should then be palpated for any subtle inconsistencies or masses. The major salivary glands should be bimanually palpated, and then saliva should be expressed from the glands to assess duct patency and flow, and saliva should be evaluated for amount, consistency, color, and floor of mouth pooling (Figure 1.4). Saliva is expressed and observed by drying the duct orifice and then palpating the gland distally to proximally until saliva flows from the orifice. The dentition and periodontium should be examined, and any removable prostheses

(a)

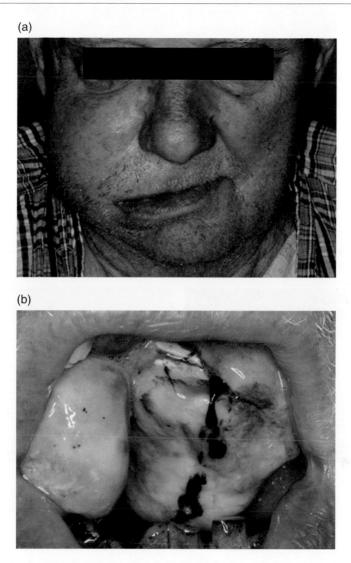

(b)

Figure 1.2   68-year-old male with notable extraoral asymmetry and swelling (a), that upon intraoral examination (b), demonstrated a large poorly differentiated carcinoma of the right maxilla.

inspected for fit and function. The oropharyngeal anatomy, and in particular the tonsils, should be assessed for symmetry, size, color, and the presence of exudates or other abnormalities that might prompt referral to an otolaryngologist for further evaluation (Figure 1.5).

1.3   Ordering and performing laboratory tests

Laboratory investigations may be necessary to determine a diagnosis or to evaluate for risk prior to dental treatment. How to order laboratory tests and, importantly, what test to order, when, why, and how to interpret the results are critical to the understanding of laboratory medical procedures. Retesting to confirm abnormal findings should always be considered, in particular when the findings are unexpected.

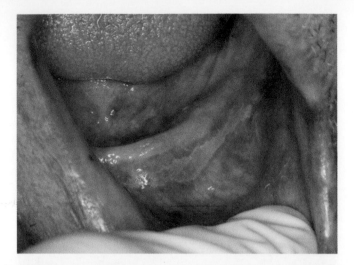

Figure 1.3 Well-defined area of leukoplakia of the anterior mandibular alveolar mucosa, with a distinct white appearance, against a background of normal-appearing pink mucosa.

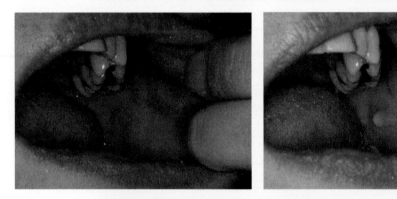

Figure 1.4 Clear aqueous saliva expressed by palpating the parotid gland extraorally.

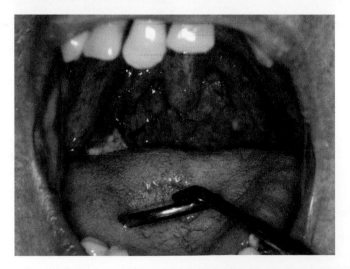

Figure 1.5 Squamous cell carcinoma of the right palatine tonsil (arrow), appearing enlarged and erythematous with extensive ulceration.

1.3.1   *Basics of ordering laboratory tests*

1.3.1.1   *Identifying a clinical laboratory*

Before a laboratory test can be ordered, a clinical laboratory must be identified. Options include a local hospital or commercial laboratory, such as Quest Diagnostics (www.questdiagnostics.com). The laboratory should be contacted regarding procedures for ordering tests, necessary supplies (e.g., culture kits), and where/how to order the recommended kits.

Alternatively, most testing can be coordinated through a patient's primary care physician. In many cases, especially for the typical oral health care provider practicing outside of a larger health care facility, collaboration with the patient's primary care physician may be the easiest option. Specific orders should be sent in writing to the physician's office and a copy of the results should be requested.

1.3.1.2   *Completion of forms*

When ordering laboratory tests, the correct requisition forms must be used and fully completed. It can be very frustrating for the provider and patient when an incorrect test is run by accident. Typically an ICD-9 code (see section 1.3.1.3) is required for each test being ordered. By law, all submitted specimens must be accompanied by two patient identifiers (e.g., name and date of birth, on both the labeled specimen and the requisition form), and when appropriate (i.e., with a biopsy or culture) the site should be specified. Questions regarding the completion of requisition forms should be directed to the clinical laboratory.

1.3.1.3   *ICD-9 codes*

The International Classification of Diseases (ICD) is a coding system created and maintained by the World Health Organization that is used for a number of purposes, including medical billing. The ICD provides a standardized classification of disease by etiology and anatomic localization. In the United States, the version that is used is the Ninth Revision, Clinical Modification, or ICD-9-CM; and this can be found on the internet or is available for purchase in print and electronic formats. Current Procedural Terminology codes, or CPT codes, are created and maintained by the American Medical Association and are used for medical billing of procedures, such as an oral biopsy. Laboratory tests and CPT codes need to have associated ICD-9 codes.

1.3.2   *Serologic studies*

Blood tests are used routinely in medicine, and in many cases may be required for evaluation of patients requiring dental care or for the work-up of patients with medical conditions affecting the oral cavity. Blood tests can be used to assess bleeding or infection risk, organ function, glucose management, and the presence of autoimmune or inflammatory diseases. The volume of blood required depends on the type and number of tests that are ordered and will be determined by the phlebotomist performing the blood collection. The main risk associated with blood collection is slight pain and bruising at the site of venipuncture. Serologic testing for specific diseases/conditions is described in greater detail throughout the clinical guide.

1.3.3   *Microbiology studies*

Microbiology studies are often necessary when evaluating a patient with suspected infection. In some cases, it may be important to identify a specific pathogen or to test for antimicrobial susceptibility so that appropriate therapy can be prescribed. The ordering clinician

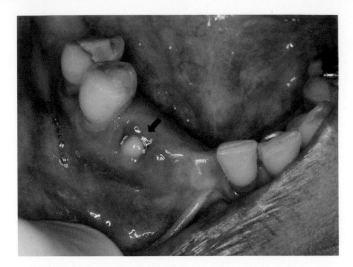

Figure 1.6 Persistent purulence despite broad-spectrum antibiotic therapy in a 50-year female with metastatic breast cancer and Stage 0 medication-associated osteonecrosis of the jaw.

must understand when to order a test, which kit to use, and any transport considerations (i.e., ice for a viral specimen). While blood, urine, and cerebrospinal fluid can all be tested microbiologically, it would be rare for an oral health professional to submit anything other than an oral specimen.

1.3.3.1 *Performing cultures*
There are several culture techniques, each with a very specific indication. Failure to use the correct technique will generally result in non-interpretable findings. As already discussed, whenever there is any question as to what test to order, and how to properly obtain and submit the sample, the clinical laboratory should be consulted directly. In addition to correctly completing the appropriate laboratory requisition form, the culture specimen should be clearly labeled with the patient's name, date of birth, date of service, and site.

1.3.3.2 *Bacterial cultures*
Bacterial culture of the oral cavity is rarely indicated except in cases of purulence (Figure 1.6). Swabbing of non-purulent mucosa will invariably demonstrate "normal oral flora." In most cases, a culture is ordered after failing initial empiric antibiotic therapy; therefore, to ensure thoroughness, both aerobic and anaerobic culture and susceptibility (sensitivity) testing should be requested. The purulence should be sampled directly, collected either by swabbing with the kit's cotton-tipped applicator, or by aspiration (in particular for anaerobic culture samples), and placed directly (cotton tip first) into the appropriate culture medium, then sealed. The susceptibility test results should ultimately guide appropriate antimicrobial therapy selection.

1.3.3.3 *Fungal cultures*
Candida albicans is the most common fungal organism in the oral cavity and is a normal component of the oral microflora in a significant proportion of the general population. It is therefore not uncommon to have a positive fungal culture in the absence of infection. Fungal cultures should only be ordered when confirmation of a diagnosis of infection is essential,

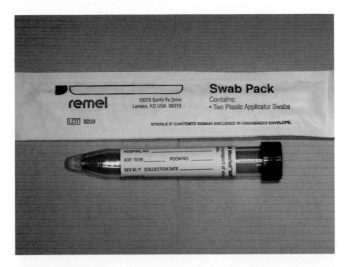

Figure 1.7 Viral culture kit.

or in situations where antifungal susceptibility testing is necessary following failure of standard empiric therapy. Using the same type of culture kit as that used for aerobic bacterial culture, the area of infection is gently swabbed with the cotton-tipped applicator provided in the kit, placed tip first into the culture medium, and sealed. Culture results should always be interpreted critically, and if a lesion has not responded to what should otherwise be adequate therapy, further susceptibility testing and/or biopsy may be indicated.

1.3.3.4 *Viral cultures*
Viral culture is highly specific, indicating that a positive result is almost always reflective of active infection. Both herpes simplex virus (HSV) and varicella zoster virus (VZV) can be readily cultured from the oral cavity. Importantly, false negatives are common; therefore, treatment for a suspected HSV infection should almost always be initiated empirically, regardless of confirmation of the diagnosis. Less commonly, false positives can be encountered due to subclinical physiologic oral shedding of virus in the absence of signs of infection.

Viral culture medium must be used and the specimen should be immediately transported to the laboratory or kept on ice when on-site facilities are not available to ensure submission of a viable specimen. Ulcerative lesions are lightly swabbed with the sterile cotton tip, which is then placed tip down into the medium and sealed (Figure 1.7). When positive, results are typically identified by the laboratory technician within the first 48 hours of culture. The direct fluorescence antibody (DFA) test is a rapid HSV test that can be useful when an immediate (same-day) diagnosis is required. DFA may also be used to confirm positive culture results, which otherwise show non-specific viral cytopathic changes, and to type HSV-1 or HSV-2. Polymerase chain reaction (PCR) is an extremely sensitive assay that is primarily used for testing of the cerebrospinal fluid in cases of viral encephalitis, and tests are available for most of the human herpes viruses. PCR is not typically used to evaluate suspected oral infections.

Cytomegalovirus (CMV) is a very rare cause of oral ulcers in immunocompromised patients. This virus cannot be cultured from the surface exudate of ulcers, as the virus is located in the endothelium and other mesenchymal cells of the connective tissue. If CMV infection is suspected, an incisional biopsy of ulcerated tissue should be obtained.

(a)

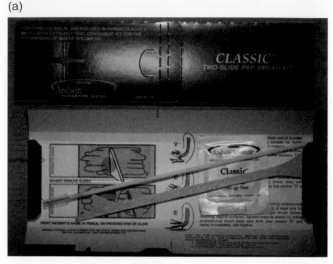

(b)

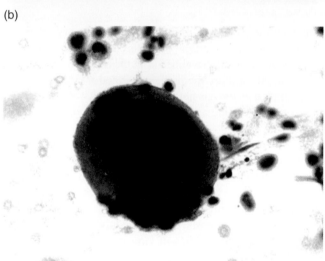

Figure 1.8 Cytology kit (a) and cytology specimen (b) demonstrating virally infected multinucleated cells, consistent with a diagnosis of herpes simplex virus infection.

1.3.3.5 *Cytopathology studies*

When an immediate diagnosis is necessary, the following cytology-based tests can be performed and interpreted in a very short period of time, depending on available resources and/ or laboratory support. Cytology specimens are obtained using either a cytology brush or wooden spatula (Figure 1.8). The lesion of interest, typically clinically suspicious for either fungal or viral infection, is gently "scraped" so that cellular material is collected that can be transferred onto a glass slide. For diagnosis of fungal infection, a potassium hydroxide (KOH) preparation may be done within minutes with the patient still in the office, while the periodic acid Schiff stain highlights fungal organisms under light microscopy (Figure 1.9). For diagnosis of herpes infection, the Tzank test, or Tzank smear, is a cytology specimen that is treated with Papanicolaou, Wright's or Giemsa stain and evaluated under a microscope for balloon-like multinucleated giant cells that are indicative of herpes virus infection.

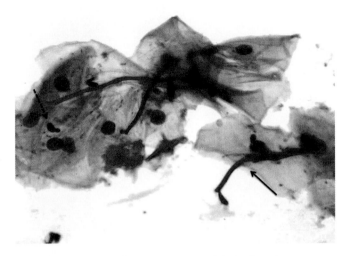

Figure 1.9 Oral cytology specimen demonstrating *Candida* hyphae (linear organisms; solid arrow) and conidiae (ovoid budding organisms; broken arrow).
Photomicrograph courtesy of Mark Lerman, DMD, Boston, MA.

1.3.4   Histopathology studies

Histopathologic analysis of a tissue biopsy is essential for definitive diagnosis of many hard and soft tissue lesions. The ability of the pathologist to interpret the histopathologic findings is limited by the tissue sample provided, so site selection and quality of the specimen are both critical factors. Since many general pathologists are not familiar with oral pathologic conditions, it is ideal to have all biopsy specimens interpreted by a board-certified oral and maxillofacial pathologist. If a local oral pathology laboratory is not available, most services will provide pre-packaged mailing kits to facilitate submission. Whenever there is any question regarding interpretation of a pathology report, or when the findings are not consistent with the expected pathology, the provider should contact the pathologist directly to discuss the case.

1.3.4.1   *Performing a biopsy*
Obtaining a tissue biopsy in most cases is a very straightforward procedure; however, several important points must be considered to ensure meaningful results. The most important aspect is determining the site of the biopsy: it is essential that the tissue is obtained from a representative area of the lesion being sampled. If the lesion is non-homogeneous—for example, a mixed red and white lesion—several representative biopsies should be considered, as malignancy may be present focally within a larger field of dysplastic changes (Figure 1.10). Each biopsy should be clearly marked (for example "A," "B," "C," etc.) and the specific site noted on the requisition form and on the label affixed to the specimen container. If the differential diagnosis includes a vesiculobullous disorder, the biopsy should be obtained from a perilesional location that includes intact epithelium (Figure 1.11). It is critical to avoid any area of ulceration, as ulcers lack epithelium and both routine histopathology and direct immunofluorescence (section 1.3.4.2) results will invariably be non-specific and inconclusive when specimens are obtained from such areas.

   In most cases, obtaining a biopsy takes no more than 5 or 10 minutes to perform. Following informed consent, a small amount of local anesthetic with epinephrine (i.e., 1–2 milliliters of 2% lidocaine with 1:50,000 or 1:100,000 epinephrine) is injected. Use of 1:50,000 concentration of epinephrine provides excellent control of bleeding; however, caution should

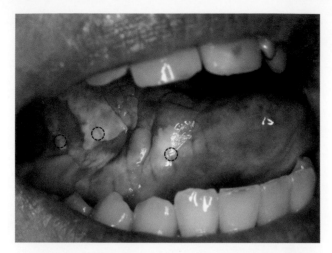

Figure 1.10 Large multifocal area of leukoplakia of the right lateral tongue in a patient already previously treated for oral squamous cell carcinoma. The three circles represent biopsy sites to obtain representative samples of the overall lesion.

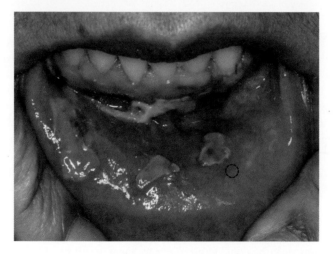

Figure 1.11 Perilesional biopsy site marked by the dashed circle that is adjacent to, but not involving, an area of ulceration.

be taken as blanching of the tissue may make definition of the lesion difficult to discern. If necessary, the biopsy site or lesion borders can be marked with a surgical pen. The mucosa should always be dried with gauze to ensure a clean and non-slippery cutting surface. For most intraoral incisional biopsies, use of a tissue punch provides a clean and easy way to obtain a sample. A 3- to 5-millimeter diameter disposable punch is rotated into the epithelium and underlying connective tissue, then removed. The specimen is grasped with tissue forceps and the deep margin is then released with scissors or a scalpel (Figure 1.12). When biopsying the attached keratinized mucosa of the gingiva or hard palate, in some cases a wedge biopsy with a scalpel may be easier than attempting to manipulate the tissue with a punch. Small, well-defined lesions such as with *fibromas* or *mucoceles* may be excised fully using a wedge or shave biopsy, as long as there is no suspicion for malignancy, as excision of malignant lesions requires histopathologically clear margins of unaffected tissue (Figure 1.13).

(a)

(b)

(c)

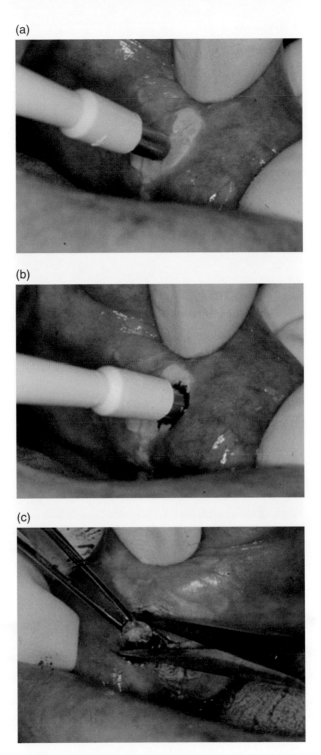

Figure 1.12 Punch biopsy sequence. The site of the biopsy is identified and the tissue punch is placed flat on the tissue (a); then the tissue punch is rotated back and forth with gentle downward pressure (b); and finally the tissue is secured with forceps, raised, and the deep base released with either scissors or a scalpel (c).

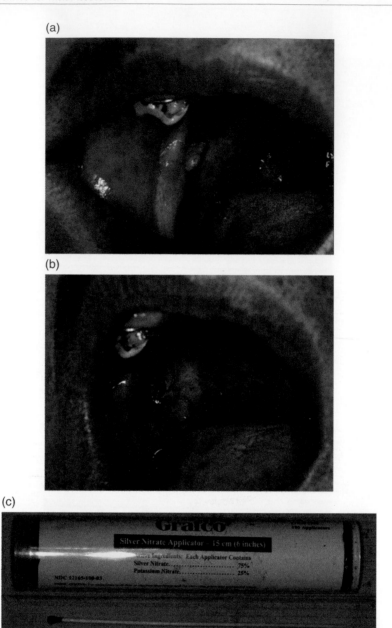

Figure 1.13 Excisional biopsy of a condyloma acuminatum of the posterior right soft palate (a, arrow). Following removal with a scalpel, silver nitrate (c) was applied to control hemostasis (b), leaving a black, cauterized wound (b).

Therefore, anytime there is suspicion for malignancy, even if the lesion could otherwise be easily excised, it is critical to first perform an incisional biopsy.

Hemostasis can be readily achieved with resorbable sutures, electrocautery, or application of silver nitrate or aluminum chloride, which causes a chemical cauterization (Figure 1.13).

Discomfort following a simple incisional biopsy is typically mild, similar to an acute bite injury, lasting for 2–3 days, and rarely requires more than over-the-counter analgesics for pain management.

1.3.4.2   *Transport medium*
The biopsy specimen must be submitted to the laboratory in a specific transport medium that is dependent upon which pathology test is required. In general, the pathology laboratory should be consulted in advance when there are any questions as to how a specimen should be properly submitted.

In most cases, specimens are placed in 10% formalin for routine histopathologic analysis. When direct immunofluorescence studies are required, in the case of a suspected autoimmune or immune-mediated vesiculobullous disorder (see chapter 11), the biopsy specimen must be submitted in either Michel's medium (preferable if the specimen will not be processed the same day of the biopsy) or saline, as formalin will fix the proteins and preclude antibody binding. Media can be ordered through a dental/medical supply company or may be provided free of charge by the oral pathology laboratory. Most immunohistochemical studies can be performed on formalin-fixed samples and are often useful in determining or refining the diagnosis; the decision to order special stains is determined by the interpreting pathologist. In rare cases, excised tissue may also be submitted for culture, in which case the specimen should be placed either in saline (for bacterial or fungal culture) or viral culture medium. Prior to submitting for culture, the microbiology laboratory should be contacted to determine the correct protocol.

1.3.4.3   *Completion of the pathology requisition form*
The requisition form is the primary means of communicating clinical information to the pathologist (Figure 1.14). While excessive and minute details are not necessary, certain key aspects of a patient's history and the clinical findings can be very useful for the pathologist when interpreting the microscopic findings. These might include any significant medical problems or exposures (e.g., tobacco, medications), a clinical description of the lesion(s) (Table 1.3), including duration and associated symptoms, biopsy location and any previous biopsy results (i.e., if a lesion previously demonstrated dysplastic changes). Photographs and/or radiographs may be submitted along with the tissue biopsy to provide the pathologist with a more complete clinical picture. For a patient with large or multifocal lesions, the biopsy site should be specified as well (e.g., anterior one-third of the right lateral tongue). The differential diagnoses should be provided, and when a specific diagnosis is suspected, this should be conveyed clearly in the appropriate section of the form.

1.3.4.4   *Interpretation of pathology results*
Pathology is not an exact science, and the same findings can be interpreted differently by different pathologists. In many cases the pathology report may be descriptive and may support a specific diagnosis; however, clinical correlation by the submitting clinician is critical in determining the correct diagnosis. It is therefore essential that the submitting provider understand the principles of histopathology and in particular how specific findings may or may not be consistent with his/her differential diagnoses. Whenever there is any question as to the meaning of the pathology report, or when the findings do not appear to be consistent with the clinical findings, the pathologist should be contacted directly to discuss the results.

BRIGHAM AND WOMEN'S HOSPITAL
A Teaching Affiliate of Harvard Medical School
75 Francis Street, Boston, Massachusetts 02115

PATHOLOGY REQUISITION

Specimen(s) will not be processed unless required fields are completed.

Location:
☐ OR
☐ Urology
☐ Interventional Radiology
☐ Endoscopy
☐ Thoracic
☐ DFCI
☐ Other
☐ Ob/Gyn
☐ Dermatology
☐ Foxboro

ORDERING PHYSICIAN: (REQUIRED) BWH Clinician ID

Print First Name Last Name

Physician Signature (Required)

Address if not BWH (Print)

** CLINICAL INFORMATION IS ABSOLUTELY REQUIRED **

Patient Information (Addressograph)
(Required)

Specimen Information

Date of Service
Required

Accession No. (by Pathology)

Path Service Requested: ☐ Gen Surg ☐ OB/Perinatal ☐ Neuro Path

CLINICAL HISTORY - INCLUDE PERTINENT LABORATORY DATA

OPERATION

OPERATIVE FINDINGS

CLINICAL DIAGNOSIS

PRE-OP.

POST-OP.

ORGAN(S) OR TISSUE(S) SUBMITTED
(Label A, B, C, etc.)

PREVIOUS SURGERY - INCLUDE DATE AND PLACE
Pathology Accession Numbers (If Known)

CHECK AS APPLICABLE
Radiation Rx ____
Chemotherapy, or
Immunosuppressive Rx ____
Hormonal Rx
Specify ________

FOR GYNECOLOGICAL CASES

LMP ________

SEND DUPLICATE REPORT TO:

Print FIRST NAME LAST NAME, M.D. Clinician ID ADDRESS IF NOT BWH (Print)

Print FIRST NAME LAST NAME, M.D. Clinician ID ADDRESS IF NOT BWH (Print)

INSTRUCTIONS

FORM MUST BE COMPLETED OR COUNTERSIGNED BY THE ORDERING PHYSICIAN OTHERWISE SPECIMEN CANNOT BE ACCEPTED.
Physician's name(s) MUST be legible and include Clinician ID.
Place BIOPSIES in Formalin. Wrap LARGE SPECIMENS in sterile, moistened Towels, place in plastic bag, or container and refrigerate.

FOR CONSULT READING ON OUTSIDE SLIDES, INCLUDE COPY OF PREVIOUS PATHOLOGY REPORTS
COMPLETE THIS FORM ON EVERY SPECIMEN AND ATTACH BILLING INFORMATION AS APPROPRIATE

0515935 (8/09)

Figure 1.14 Typical pathology requisition form. In addition to the required information at the top of the page, the clinician should provide sufficient clinical details such as the size, location, and appearance of the lesion. Used with permission from Brigham and Women's Hospital.

1.4 Radiology studies

Oral health care providers in some ways function as specialized dental radiologists since most practitioners obtain and interpret their own intraoral and panoramic radiographs. While oral health care providers rarely order other imaging studies of the head and neck, it is

Table 1.3   Clinical descriptors of oral lesions.

Category	Term	Description
Size, shape, thickness	Atrophy	Loss of tissue, typically due to thinning of cell layers; often associated with erythema clinically
	Bulla	A fluid-filled blister > 0.5 cm in diameter
	Endophytic	A lesion that appears to be growing inward, toward the underlying tissues
	Erosion	Loss or thinning of superficial epithelial layers not extending through the full thickness of epithelium, typically secondary to inflammation; appears red
	Exophytic	A lesion that appears to be growing outward from the surface
	Macule	A flat lesion defined by color or texture changes
	Papillary	A lesion with multiple finger-like projections
	Papule	A well-defined elevated lesion < 0.5 cm in diameter
	Plaque	A well-defined elevated lesion > 0.5 cm in diameter
	Pustule	A small, well-defined accumulation of pus, usually located superficially
	Ulcer	Complete loss of epithelium, typically presenting with a yellow or whitish-grey pseudomembrane
	Vegetation	An exophytic lesion with multiple papillary or nodular areas of outgrowth
	Verrucous	Papillary and deeply folded epithelial changes that can appear wart-like or wrinkled
	Vesicle	A fluid-filled blister < 0.5 cm in diameter
Color, pigment, vascular	Ecchymosis	A macular area of submucosal hemorrhage ("bruise") appearing as a well-defined area of erythema or purplish-blue pigmentation
	Erythema	Redness of the mucosa secondary to increased vascularity and/or epithelial atrophy
	Hematoma	A collection of blood in the connective tissue presenting as a well-defined raised red, purple, or black lesion
	Leukoplakia	A white lesion that does not rub away and that cannot be defined by any obvious clinical entity
	Petechia	A small, punctate area of submucosal hemorrhage
Findings upon palpation	Fixed	A lesion that is non-mobile and firmly attached to the underlying structures
	Indurated	Hard, firm tissue that would normally be soft
	Mobile	A freely movable lesion that does not appear to be attached to underlying structures
	Nodule	A solid mass visible or palpable within or underneath the mucosa
	Pedunculated	An exophytic lesion attached to the mucosa by a thinner stalk
	Sessile	An exophytic lesion that is firmly attached to the mucosa by a broad base

important that they be familiar with the various available imaging modalities and how they are used throughout the field of medicine. When pathology is suspected that requires an advanced imaging study, the patient should be referred to his/her primary care physician for ordering such studies. When available, patients may also be referred for evaluation by a board-certified oral and maxillofacial radiologist. There should always be a clear indication for ordering radiographic studies, either to contribute to diagnosis, to guide management, or to assess response to therapy.

1.4.1   *Plain film*

Intraoral periapical and bitewing radiographs are the gold standard for imaging the dentition. Panoramic radiography provides an acceptable image of the mandible and maxilla and is useful in evaluating any bony lesions of the jaws, though it is important to recognize the limitations

(a)

(b)

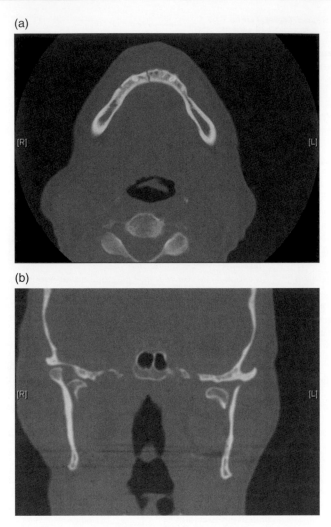

Figure 1.15 Computed tomography of the mandible in a trauma patient. Axial view (a) demonstrates a symphisis fracture and the coronal view (b) demonstrates bilateral condylar head fractures.

of visualizing three-dimensional structures on two-dimensional films. While not optimal for evaluating the teeth, a panoramic radiograph can be sufficient, at least for assessment of gross dental pathology, for patients in whom it is not possible to obtain intraoral images. Maxillary and mandibular occlusal films are used for imaging the palate and floor of mouth.

1.4.2 Computed tomography

Computed tomography (CT) provides excellent high resolution hard tissue imaging. With certain limitations, soft tissues can also be visualized with the use of intravenous contrast agent; however, magnetic resonance imaging (MRI) provides much greater soft tissue imaging resolution (section 1.4.3). In the head and neck region, CT is utilized to determine location, size, and extent of lesions; evaluate salivary gland pathology; assess for enlarged/necrotic lymph nodes; and evaluate extent of infections (Figure 1.15). The use of cone beam

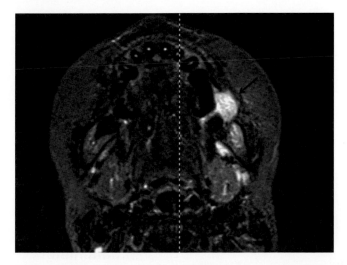

Figure 1.16 Magnetic resonance imaging of the mandible in a patient with squamous cell carcinoma of the left posterior buccal vestibule demonstrating a large enhancing lesion (tumor, arrow) that does not appear to be invading into the alveolar bone.

CT is becoming increasingly popular in dental imaging, in particular for treatment planning of dental implants. This imaging modality provides high-quality three dimensional imaging of a limited field within the head and neck at a lower radiation dose compared with traditional CT. Depending on what tissue is being studied, the radiologist may determine that a contrast agent, given intravenously just prior to the study, is required to better delineate the type of tissue and extent of associated changes.

1.4.3   Magnetic resonance imaging

MRI offers the highest resolution soft tissue imaging, and unlike CT, does not utilize ionizing radiation. Compared with CT (with contrast), MRI has a much greater ability to differentiate between different types of soft tissue. When indicated, MRI provides optimal imaging of neoplasms (location, extent, invasion into other structures) and the soft tissues of the temporomandibular joint complex, which can be visualized in both open and closed images (Figure 1.16). With T1-weighted images, fat tissue appears bright, or enhanced, whereas water and other fluids appear bright in T2-weighted images. While a brain MRI would rarely be ordered by a dentist, this diagnostic study may be utilized to rule-out central lesions that might present with orofacial manifestations (see Figure 9.2). Disadvantages of MRI include the increased time and expense (relative to CT) and the enclosed space, although "open" MRI machines are available for patients who suffer from claustrophobia.

1.4.4   Other imaging studies

Several other diagnostic modalities are available for imaging the head and neck; however, few of these are still used on any regular basis since the introduction of CT, MRI, and positron emission tomography (PET). Sialography is a salivary gland imaging technique in which a radiopaque solution is injected into the major salivary gland duct orifice to evaluate for obstructive and degenerative changes deep in the gland by noting where the dye perfuses

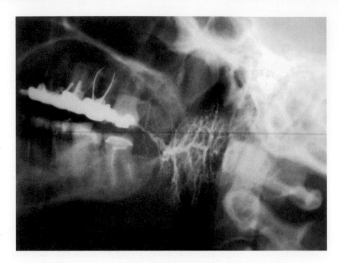

Figure 1.17   Sialogram of the parotid gland demonstrating the ductal system with loss of normal acinar structures.

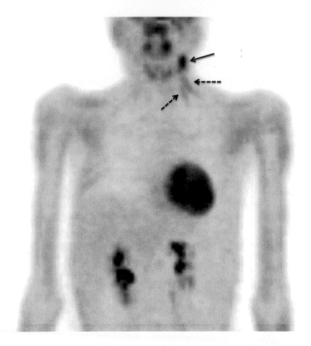

Figure 1.18   Positron emission tomography scan of the same patient from Figure 1.16, demonstrating the tumor in the left posterior mandible (arrow) as well as involvement of lymph nodes in the left neck (broken arrows).

and accumulates (Figure 1.17; see chapter 8). Scintigraphy utilizes radioisotopes that are taken up by the salivary glands and can be used to assess glandular function (see chapter 8). The use of scintigraphy is limited to research investigations.

PET scanning measures areas of increased metabolic activity and bone deposition and is used extensively for the diagnosis and surveillance of certain cancers (Figure 1.18).

(a)

(b)

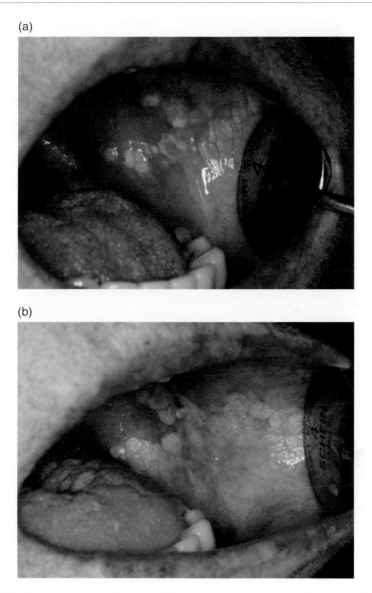

Figure 1.19 Extensive area of leukoplakia in a patient that had previously undergone allogeneic hematopoietic cell transplantation. Photographs obtained at 6 (a) and 8 (b) years post-transplantation demonstrate clear progression of the lesion. Biopsies at both visits demonstrated hyperkeratosis only.

In many cases PET and CT are combined (PET/CT) so that the PET findings can be precisely localized anatomically. Ultrasonography can be used to image soft tissue, such as the salivary glands (see chapter 8), but requires an experienced radiologist to interpret the results. Intraoral photography should be utilized to document oral soft tissue lesions and can be particularly useful for following changes over time (Figure 1.19).

1.5 Suggested literature

Dworin AM. A course in physical, clinical, and laboratory diagnosis for dental education. J Dent Educ 1979 Dec;43:685–687.

Jordan RC, Daniels TE, Greenspan JS, et al. Advanced diagnostic methods in oral and maxillofacial pathology. Part 1: Molecular methods. Oral Surg Oral Med Oral Pathol Oral Radiol Endod 2001;92: 650–669.

Jordan RC, Daniels TE, Greenspan JS, et al. Advanced diagnostic methods in oral and maxillofacial pathology. Part 2: Immunohistochemical and immunofluorescent methods. Oral Surg Oral Med Oral Pathol Oral Radiol Endod 2002;93:56–74.

Orel S, Sterrett G, Whitaker D. Fine Needle Aspiration Cytology, 4th ed. New York: Elsevier, 2005.

Shintaku W, Enciso R, Broussard J, Clark GT. Diagnostic imaging for chronic orofacial pain, maxillofacial osseous and soft tissue pathology and temporomandibular disorders. J Calif Dent Assoc 2006;34: 633–644.

World Health Organization International Classification of Diseases. http://www.who.int/classifications/icd/en/, accessed February 1, 2012.

2 Basic Tests and Evaluation Methods of Systemic Health

2.0 INTRODUCTION

Physical health indicators can provide useful information about the systemic health of patients. Some of the most basic physical assessment measures are vital signs, which should be performed routinely in the dental setting. Testing vitals can corroborate findings from the health history or identify conditions that may need to be further evaluated by medical professionals. For example, taking the blood pressure and pulse at the beginning of a dental appointment can identify patients at risk for hypertension who may need to be referred to a physician for further assessment and management. Other testing measures involve blood sampling, which may be indicated in the dental setting in certain circumstances, such as evaluating the risk for bleeding prior to a surgical procedure. Assessment of a blood glucose level in a diabetic patient may prompt modifications in the planned dental appointment to prevent a hypoglycemic episode. Since dental patients are typically seen at routine intervals, oral health care providers can play an active role in monitoring physical health measures of their patients and can encourage follow-up with medical personnel when indicated.

Basic blood measurements are useful screening tools for systemic disease. These tests involve assessment of cells, chemistry values, and electrolytes in blood and can provide information pertaining to diagnosis and monitoring of disease. Tests of red and white blood cells may be indicators of anemias and the body's ability to fight infection. Serum chemistry and electrolyte analytes provide insight regarding kidney and liver function, acid-base and fluid balance, nutritional and endocrine status, and pH homeostasis. Test results can alert the oral health care practitioner regarding potential for bleeding, infection, and systemic function, so it is important to become familiar with these clinical investigations. This chapter will introduce basic health indicators that serve as proxy measures of systemic function and will guide the oral health care provider in ordering and interpreting the results as they relate to physiologic function.

2.1 Vital signs

Vital signs include respiratory rate, temperature, pulse, blood pressure, and height and weight are recorded as part of a routine physical examination. Vital signs can serve as screening tools for systemic disease and provide baseline measures of body function. It is good practice

Risk Assessment and Oral Diagnostics in Clinical Dentistry, First Edition.
Dena J. Fischer, Nathaniel S. Treister and Andres Pinto.
© 2013 John Wiley & Sons, Inc. Published 2013 by John Wiley & Sons, Inc.

to take vital signs at new patient visits and record pulse and blood pressure at recall appointments. Assessment of the respiratory rate is usually not necessary in the dental setting unless cardiopulmonary disease is suspected or sedation is planned. The respiratory rate is determined by counting the number of times the chest rises and falls for 30 seconds. A normal rate is 12–15 respirations per minute. Measurement of a patient's temperature may be warranted when an infection is suspected. Normal body temperature is 98.6°F (37°C), and an elevated temperature indicates a systemic illness or infection.

Radial or *carotid artery pulse* is a measure of cardiac rate, rhythm, and strength. Carotid pulse is obtained using the first two fingers in the region of the carotid bulb, just below the angle of the mandible and anterior to the sternocleidomastoid muscle. Alternatively, radial pulse can be determined by placing the fingers between the radius and flexor tendons on the ventral wrist. The pulse rate is determined by counting the number of beats for 15 seconds. Normal heart rate is 60–80 beats per minute (bpm). A high pulse (greater than 100 bpm) is tachycardia and may be an indicator of a cardiac condition, while a low pulse (less than 60 bpm) is bradycardia (Alert Box 2.1). The *pulse rhythm* refers to the pattern of the beats. In a regular pulse rhythm, the time between beats is constant, while an irregular rhythm does not have an even pattern and can signify an abnormal cardiac condition, such as an arrhythmia or atrial fibrillation. An intermittent pulse is an irregular rhythm in which the beat is missed at regular or irregular intervals. Finally, the *pulse strength* (force) is an indicator of the amount of blood forced into the artery by the heartbeat. A normal pulse has normal strength. A very strong or bounding pulse occurs when the heart is pumping a large amount of blood with each heartbeat. This can occur normally with heavy exercise, high anxiety, or alcohol consumption, or it could be a sign of a cardiac abnormality. A strong pulse is stronger than

Alert Box 2.1 Reference ranges for radial or carotid artery pulse.

Risk level	Pulse rate Number of beats per minute (bpm)	Pulse rhythm Pattern of heartbeats	Pulse strength Indicator of amount of blood pumped into artery with each heartbeat
Low (normal)	60–80 bpm (resting pulse)	Time between beats is constant	Normal pulse strength
Moderate	*High/low values* Tacchycardia: 80–100 bpm Bradychardia: < 60 bpm	*Irregular* Irregular pattern of beats; may indicate arrhythmia or atrial fibrillation	*Strong pulse* Heart is pumping large amount of blood with each heartbeat; may occur with exercise or can indicate cardiac abnormality
		Intermittent Beat is missed at regular or irregular intervals	*Weak pulse* Heart is pumping small amount of blood with each heartbeat
High	*High value* Severe tacchycardia: > 100 bpm*	N/A	*Bounding pulse* Extremely strong pulse; may occur with shock or severe hemorrhage

* If not associated with exercise/physical exertion.

Table 2.1   Classification of hypertension.*,†

Category	Systolic blood pressure (mm Hg)	Diastolic blood pressure (mm Hg)
Normal	< 120	and < 80
Pre-hypertension	120–139	or 80–89
Hypertension Stage 1	140–159	or 90–99
Hypertension Stage 2	≥ 160	or ≥ 100
Isolated systolic hypertension	≥ 140	and < 90

*Medical management using antihypertensive drugs is recommended at or above hypertension Stage 1. In patients with chronic kidney disease or diabetes, medical management is recommended if blood pressure is ≥ 130/80 mm Hg.
†Adapted from National Heart, Lung and Blood Institute, National Institutes of Health, U.S. Department of Health and Human Services. The Seventh Report of the Joint National Committee on Prevention, Detection, Evaluation and Treatment of High Blood Pressure. NIH Publication, December 2003.

a normal pulse, but is less than bounding and may occur with shock or severe hemorrhage. A weak pulse is hard to detect and indicates that the heart is pumping only a small amount of blood with each heartbeat.

Blood pressure assesses pressure within the arteries during cardiac contraction (*systole*) and cardiac pause (*diastole*). This is measured using a manual or electronic sphygmoma-nometer placed around the upper arm. The pressure generated by the cuff exceeds that within the arteries and is slowly released to detect the pulse as blood is again pumped through the vessels. The pressure at which the first evidence of a pulse is detected is the systolic, and the pressure at which a pulse can no longer be detected is the diastolic. The *auscultatory gap* is the interval of pressure where sounds indicating systolic pressure fade away and reappear at a lower pressure point during the manual measurement of blood pressure. Improper interpretation of this gap may lead to an underestimation of systolic blood pressure and/or an overestimation of diastolic readings. It is therefore recommended to palpate the radial artery and inflate the blood pressure cuff until the radial artery pulse disappears to obtain the true systolic pressure when manually recording a patient's blood pressure.

Blood pressure values are a standard screening tool for hypertension, and the Seventh Report of the Joint National Committee (JNC7) has developed a simple classification system for blood pressure levels and categories of hypertension (Table 2.1). A systolic or diastolic blood pressure measurement higher than the accepted normal values (less than 120/80 mm Hg) is classified as *pre-hypertension* (120–139/80–89 mm Hg) or *hypertension* (140/90 mm Hg or greater). Isolated systolic hypertension refers to elevated systolic pressure with normal diastolic pressure and is common in older adults. Individuals with blood pressures 130/80 mm Hg or greater with concomitant diabetes mellitus or chronic kidney disease are classified as having hypertension. Patients on whom abnormal blood pressure readings are detected should be referred to a physician for further evaluation and management. Medical management with antihypertensive medication is recommended for all patients with hypertension (as specified in JNC7), and dental procedures should be delayed in patients with uncontrolled Stage 2 hypertension since these individuals are at increased risk for cardiac events, such as myocardial infarction and/or cerebrovascular accident.

Oxygen saturation is a percentage indicating the ratio between the actual oxygen content of hemoglobin (Hgb) and the potential maximum oxygen-carrying capacity of Hgb. It is determined using a pulse oximeter, a small, clip-like sensor that is placed on a digit over the fingernail. Normal levels range from 95% to 100%. Oxygen level below 86% requires emergency medical intervention (i.e., administer oxygen, send to urgent care facility or emergency room). Measuring oxygen saturation in the dental environment is mandatory when sedation is used to monitor breathing, and may be considered during surgical procedures, particularly in patients with medical conditions that can cause hypoxia (e.g., chronic obstructive pulmonary disorder, emphysema, congestive heart failure).

2.2   Diagnostic fluids

2.2.1   Blood

Blood is the most commonly used diagnostic fluid, particularly because it is obtained in a simple, relatively non-invasive manner and has tremendous potential for basic screening, diagnosis, and monitoring of disease. Blood is typically drawn through venipuncture, in which an adequate volume of venous blood can be obtained for most laboratory tests. Capillary puncture (skin puncture) may be performed when smaller quantities of blood are sufficient. *Whole blood* is composed of blood cells suspended in a liquid called blood plasma. *Plasma* is mostly water and also contains dissolved proteins, electrolytes (mainly sodium and chloride ions), blood-clotting factors, hormones, glucose, and carbon dioxide. The *blood cells* present in blood are white cells (*leukocytes*), red cells (*erythrocytes*), and platelets (*thrombocytes*). The term *serum* refers to plasma from which the clotting proteins have been removed. Most of the proteins remaining in serum are albumin and immunoglobulins (antibodies). Blood tests can screen for systemic disease and dysfunction (e.g., diabetes, kidney/liver dysfunction), certain blood disorders (e.g., anemia, leukemia), abnormal bleeding and clotting (e.g., hemophilia, thrombocytopenia), inflammation (e.g., autoimmune disorders) and infection (e.g., HIV).

2.2.2   Saliva as a diagnostic fluid

Point-of-care (POC) diagnostics refers to tests performed in the primary care setting to provide results rapidly and accelerate clinical decision making. Some advantages of using saliva for POC testing include non-invasive collection, possibility for self-collection, and the fact that salivary levels of many molecules reflect that in blood and urine, though in lower concentrations. Perhaps the most widespread use of these tests is the oral fluid-based test for antibodies to HIV. This test is safe and easy to use, though positive results should be confirmed with serum tests. Saliva can also be used to identify and monitor the presence of chemicals and molecules used in the health care setting such as drugs (illicit, over-the-counter, prescription), steroid hormones, and tobacco (see chapter 8).

Researchers are studying the potential of using saliva to diagnose oral and systemic conditions. The presence of antibodies in saliva may aid with the diagnosis of other infectious diseases such as hepatitis and bacterial infections, and proteins, hormones, and RNA transcripts in saliva may be associated with certain cancers, including oral, breast, and ovarian cancer. In addition, specific inflammatory mediators and enzymes in saliva may serve as biomarkers for the diagnosis of oral disease such as periodontitis and dental caries as well as systemic disease such as acute myocardial infarction. The field of salivary diagnostics is emerging research, and in the future saliva may contribute to POC diagnosis of numerous oral and systemic conditions as well as monitoring health and response to treatment.

Table 2.2   Complete blood count (CBC) tests.

Test	Conventional abbreviation	Clinical significance of values
White blood cell count	WBC	Ability to fight infection; hematologic dysfunction or malignancy; presence of infection (leukocytosis) or allergy (eosinophilia)
Differential white blood cell count	Diff	Specific patterns of WBCs; type of infection; ability to fight infection
Red blood cell count	RBC	Ability to carry oxygen from lungs to blood tissues and carbon dioxide from tissue to lungs; anemia
Hematocrit	Hct	RBC mass
Hemoglobin	Hgb	Main component of RBCs; ability to transport oxygen and carbon dioxide
Red blood cell indices – Mean corpuscular volume – Mean corpuscular hemoglobin concentration – Mean corpuscular hemoglobin Stained red cell examination – Red blood cell distribution width – Reticulocyte %	 MCV MCHC MCH RDW Retic %	Diagnosis of anemias Hct% x 10/RBC Hgb x 100/Hct% Hgb x 10/RBC SD of RBC size x 100/MCV Total retic/,1000 RBCs x 100
Platelet count	Plt	Ability to clot and control bleeding
Mean platelet volume	MPV	Uniformity of platelet size

SD = standard deviation.

2.2.3   Other diagnostic fluids

Urine is composed of urea and other organic and inorganic waste products and can provide information about the body's major metabolic functions. It is readily available and easily collected, so urinalysis can be a valuable metabolic screening procedure. Stool studies may be helpful in diagnosing gastrointestinal disorders. Cerebrospinal fluid (CSF) is a clear fluid formed within the ventricles of the brain, which circulates from the ventricles into the space surrounding the brain and spinal cord, helping to regulate intracranial pressure, supply nutrients to tissues, and remove waste products. Most CSF constituents are present in the same or lower concentrations as in the blood plasma; however, disease can cause elements typically restrained by the blood-brain barrier to enter the spinal fluid. CSF can be obtained by lumbar puncture and is the main diagnostic tool for neurologic disorders such as meningitis, subarachnoid hemorrhage, CNS malignancy, and multiple sclerosis.

2.3   General blood tests

The complete blood count (CBC) is a basic screening tool and is one of the most frequently ordered laboratory tests. The findings in the CBC give valuable diagnostic information about the hematologic and other body systems, prognosis, and response to treatment. The CBC consists of a series of tests that determine number, variety, percentage, concentrations, and quality of each of the basic types of blood cells (Table 2.2). The shorthand notation for common hematology values is illustrated in Figure 2.1.

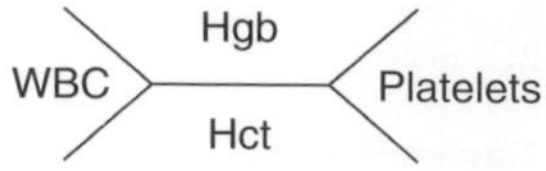

Figure 2.1   Shorthand notation for common hematology values.

2.3.1   Hematopoiesis

Hematopoiesis is the production and differentiation of blood cells from hematopoietic stem cells. Stem cells reside in the bone marrow and have the ability to give rise to all types of blood cells (multipotency), and they also have the capacity to self-renew. Hematopoietic stem cells differentiate into two lineages of cells, myeloid and lymphoid progenitor cells. With the aid of growth factors, these cells proliferate and mature into their end product blood cells. Numerous growth factors stimulate and regulate the production of all types of leukocytes (white blood cells). Erythropoietin, a growth factor secreted into the bloodstream by renal tubular epithelium, is required for a myeloid progenitor cell to become an erythrocyte (red blood cell), and thrombopoietin is a growth factor produced by the liver and kidney that regulates production of thrombocytes (platelets).

2.3.2   Red blood cells

The main function of erythrocytes is to carry oxygen from the lungs to the body tissues and to transfer carbon dioxide from the tissues to the lungs. The average lifespan of the erythrocyte is 120 days. Hgb is the main component of the red blood cell (RBC) and serves to carry the oxygen and carbon dioxide. The RBC is shaped like a biconcave disk to provide more surface area for the Hgb to combine with oxygen.

Hgb is synthesized in erythroblasts (immature red blood cells) and requires folic acid and vitamin B_{12} for full maturation. The Hgb molecule is a complex structure that is comprised of a heme (porphyrin) ring with ferric ions and protein components. When erythrocytes are broken down, the heme ring of the Hgb is transformed to bilirubin and metabolized through the liver (therefore, increased bilirubin is an indicator of liver dysfunction; section 2.4.1), and the iron is recycled back into newly generated erythrocytes.

2.3.2.1   Basic tests of red blood cells

Anemia occurs when there is decreased Hgb, caused by a reduction in the number of circulating erythrocytes, the amount of Hgb (an indirect measure of cell mass), and/or the volume of packed cells (hematocrit [Hct]). Since the RBC, Hgb, and Hct counts are closely related, these values are typically evaluated together as part of the CBC, and reference values are presented in Alert Box 2.2. Hct is expressed as the percentage by volume of packed RBCs in whole blood. Hgb concentration is important in evaluation of anemia since the oxygen-carrying capacity of blood is directly proportional to the Hgb concentration rather than the RBC because some RBCs contain more Hgb than others. Hgb also serves a role of adjusting the pH of the extracellular fluid and therefore alternately binding with oxygen or carbon dioxide. A severely low Hct or Hgb can lead to cardiac failure and death (due to decreased oxygen-carrying capacity to tissues), while a severely high Hct or Hgb is associated with spontaneous blood clotting (due to an increase in RBC mass and blood viscosity).

Polycythemia is an abnormal increase in RBC, Hct, and/or Hgb and is classified as: (a) *absolute*, where there is an increase in RBC mass, or (b) *relative*, in which the RBC mass

Alert Box 2.2   RBC value reference ranges and restrictions/modifications for dental treatment.

Risk level	RBCs (cells/mm³)	Hct (%)	Hgb (g/dL)	Interventions
Low (normal in males)	$4.2–5.4 \times 10^6$	42–52	14.0–17.4	None
Low (normal in females)	$3.6–5.0 \times 10^6$	3–48	12.0–16.0	None
Moderate	More accurate to assess Hct, Hgb	50–69 (high) 21–40 (low)	16–20 (high) 8–12 (low)	None
High	More accurate to assess Hct, Hgb	> 60 (high)	> 20 (high)	High: Obtain medical consultation, spontaneous clotting may occur
		< 20 (low)	< 8 (low)	Low: Obtain medical consultation, avoid elective surgical procedures, limit narcotic use

is normal with a decreased plasma volume. Absolute primary polycthemia may occur with the myeloproliferative disorder *polycythemia vera* as well as *erythremic erythrocytosis*, a condition in which increased RBC production occurs in the bone marrow. Absolute secondary polycythemia may develop due to an increase in erythropoietin secretion in response to hypoxia, as with pulmonary or cardiovascular disease, renal tumors, or a physiologic response to high altitude. Relative polycythemia may occur during dehydration, resulting from a decrease in plasma volume.

2.3.2.2   *Red blood cell indices*

The RBC indices define the size and Hgb content of the RBC and are used to classify and differentiate anemias based upon RBC size (normocytic, macrocytic, microcytic) and Hgb concentration, which affects color (normochromic, hyperchromic, hypochromic; Table 2.3). The results of indices are ascertained with a peripheral blood smear, which is used to assess RBC morphology (RBC size and Hgb content).

The *mean corpuscular volume* (MCV) is the volume occupied by a single erythrocyte, measured in cubic micrometers of the average red blood cell volume, and is an indicator of RBC size. The *mean corpuscular hemoglobin concentration* (MCHC) measures the average concentration of Hgb in the RBCs. Decreased MCHC values signify that a unit volume of packed RBCs contains less Hgb than normal, and the cells are hypochromic. *Mean corpuscular hemoglobin* (MCH) is a measure of the average weight of Hgb per RBC and contributes to cell size in severely anemic patients. The *red cell size distribution width* (RDW) is an indicator of the degree of abnormal variation in size of RBCs and can help to differentiate between some types of anemias. Increased RDW occurs in iron-deficiency anemia, pernicious anemia, and immune hemolytic anemia, while normal RDW may be found with aplastic anemia and sickle cell disease. *Platelet count* and other platelet function tests are used to diagnose platelet disorders and are discussed in chapter 3.

Table 2.3 Classification of anemias.

Anemia classification	Disorder/pathophysiology	Example
Microcytic, hypochromic	Disorders of iron metabolism	Iron-deficiency anemia Plummer-Vinson syndrome
	Disorders of globin synthesis	Thalassemias Sickle cell disease
Normocytic, normochromic	Anemia with appropriate bone marrow response Anemia with impaired bone marrow response	Acute post-hemorrhagic anemia G6PD deficiency Aplastic anemia Decreased erythropoietin production
Macrocytic, hyperchromic	Vitamin B_{12} deficiency	Pernicious anemia Decreased dietary intake Impaired absorption
	Folate deficiency	Decreased dietary intake Impaired absorption

G6PD = Glucose-6-phosphate dehydrogenase.

2.3.2.3 *Other RBC tests*

The *erythrocyte sedimentation rate* (ESR) is the rate at which erythrocytes settle out of anticoagulated blood in 1 hour. This test is based on the fact that inflammatory and necrotic processes cause an alteration in blood proteins, resulting in aggregation of RBCs, which makes them heavier and more likely to fall rapidly when placed in a special vertical test tube. The faster the settling of the cells, the higher the ESR value. It is not diagnostic for any particular disease, but elevated levels indicate an inflammatory disease process that needs to be investigated further. Normal ESR values range from 0 to 20 mm/h for adults and 0 to 30 mm/h for adults over age 50.

2.3.2.4 *Anemias*

Clinically, anemia results in tissues supplied by the circulation receiving a deficient quantity of oxygen, and general symptoms include pallor of the skin, conjunctiva, and nail beds; dyspnea; and fatigue. Pallor of oral mucosal tissues and loss of filiform papillae (smooth, red tongue) may be evident as anemia progresses (Figures 2.2 and 2.3). In general, anemias do not pose a serious risk for patients seeking dental care unless general anesthetics are to be administered. Extremely low hemoglobin levels (less than 8 g/dL) may be associated with decreased RBC production, hemolysis of RBCs, or blood loss. In these patients, elective surgical procedures should be avoided since there is a potential for clinical bleeding and faulty wound healing. Narcotic use should also be limited for those with severe anemia due to the potential for hypoxia secondary to decreased oxygen-carrying capacity to tissues.

2.3.2.4.1 *Vitamin and mineral deficiencies*

The most common cause of anemia is iron deficiency, caused by chronic blood loss or a deficiency of dietary iron. Since iron is necessary for the production of Hgb, this deficiency results in a microcytic, hypochromic anemia with decreased numbers of RBCs. Diagnosis can be determined with RBC indices, which reveal a decreased MCV, MCHC, and MCH, and microcytic, hypochromic cells are present on a peripheral blood smear. In addition, serum iron and ferritin concentrations are reduced. Normal serum iron (Fe) concentration

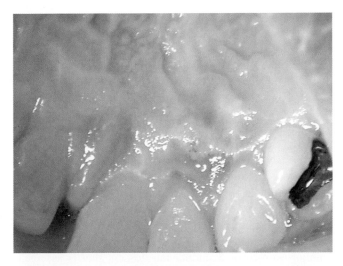

Figure 2.2 Pallor of the palate in a 41-year-old female with pernicious anemia.

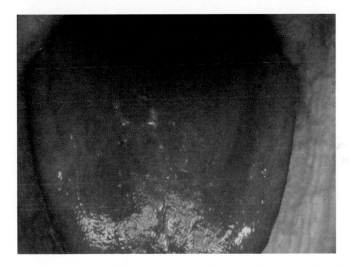

Figure 2.3 Tongue pallor and loss of filiform papillae in a 36-year-old female with iron deficiency anemia.

levels in adults are 65–175 μg/dL for men and 50–170 μg/dL for women. Ferritin is a complex of ferric hydroxide and apoferritin and is the most reliable indicator of total-body iron status. Ferritin is a very sensitive test for diagnosing iron deficiency because it decreases before anemia and other changes occur. Normal ferritin levels are 20–250 ng/mL in men and 10–120 ng/mL in women. Decreased ferritin (less than 10 ng/mL) usually indicates iron-deficiency anemia, which can be reversed by adding adequate levels of iron to the diet.

Both folic acid and vitamin B_{12} are required for erythroblastic differentiation and maturation. Folic acid is present in most foods in a well-balanced diet, and vitamin B_{12} is obtained from ingestion of animal protein. A folic acid dietary deficiency or vitamin B_{12} dietary or absorption deficiency results in megaloblastic anemia, with decreased numbers of large (macrocytic), normochromic, immature, and dysfunctional RBCs. Vitamin B_{12} absorption deficiency secondary to atrophic gastritis and loss of intrinsic factor is also known as *pernicious anemia*. Diagnosis of megaloblastic anemia is determined with elevated levels of MCV and MCH and normal MCHC. Anemia due to vitamin B_{12} deficiency develops with levels less than 100 pg/mL (normal vitamin B_{12} levels are 200–835 pg/mL). To diagnose pernicious anemia, the Schilling test is used, in which radioactive vitamin B_{12} is ingested and excreted amounts are quantified to determine absorption levels. Elevated serum homocysteine (greater than 13 μmol/L) and methylmalonic acid (greater than 0.4 μmol/L) levels may also be indicators of vitamin B_{12} deficiency. However, while these serum levels are sensitive they are not specific, as up to 25% of older adults have elevated levels of homocysteine or methylmalonic acid without B_{12} deficiency. Folic acid deficiency is confirmed with RBC indices indicating megaloblastic anemia and reduced serum levels of folic acid (normal serum folic acid levels are 2–20 ng/mL). Folic acid deficiency can be corrected by dietary supplementation, and vitamin B_{12} deficiency may require dietary supplementation if insufficient intake or injection in cases of the absorption defect.

Oral manifestations of pernicious anemia involve loss of filiform and often fungiform papillae, giving the tongue dorsum a smooth, red appearance, known as *atrophic glossitis*. Iron deficiency among women of Scandinavian descent that is associated with atrophic changes in the upper aerodigestive tract mucosa is *Plummer-Vinson syndrome*, and the atrophic mucosa is prone to transformation to squamous cell carcinomas.

2.3.2.4.2 *Hemolytic anemias*

Hemolytic anemias result from decreased survival of erythrocytes, often due to inherited enzyme deficiencies or defects of Hgb or RBC structure. These defects in Hgb structure are known as *hemoglobinopathies*, the most common of which are sickle cell disease and the thalassemias. Common diagnostic findings for hemolytic anemias are decreased MCHC and MCH values, increased reticulocyte count, and increases in serum bilirubin (section 2.4.1). Reticulocytes are immature erythrocytes, and when they account for greater than 2% of total erythrocytes, indicate an increased reticulocyte count. Abnormal Hgb proteins are detected through Hgb electrophoresis, which matches hemolyzed RBC material against standard bands for various Hgb types. Signs and symptoms of hemolytic anemia are similar to other forms of anemia (e.g., dyspnea, fatigue); however, the breakdown of RBCs may also lead to jaundice and may increase the risk of long-term complications such as gallstones and pulmonary hypertension.

Sickle cell anemia is a hereditary blood disorder in which individuals produce an abnormal Hgb, called Hgb S, that causes RBCs to take on a crescent or "sickle" shape. These deformed cells are lysed, resulting in chronic anemia. This autosomal recessive disorder is due to a single basepoint mutation in the Hgb gene and may present as a sickle cell trait (heterozygous pattern) or sickle cell anemia (homozygous pattern). Heterozygous carriers usually do not show any ill effects, but the homozygous state is associated with considerable morbidity and mortality. Sickle cell disease more commonly affects individuals of African descent. During severe episodes (sickle cell crisis), the sickled erythrocytes may occlude vessels, thereby preventing blood circulation and potentially damaging tissues and organs. Oral manifestations of sickle cell anemia include jaundice and pallor of oral tissues resulting from the anemia and hemolytic process as well as localized soft tissue and bony necrosis (infarcts; Figure 2.4) or neuropathic pain symptoms (see chapter 12) secondary to vascular occlusion. Radiographically, a "stepladder" trabeculation may be seen on dental bitewings, and skull films yield a "hair-on-end" effect due to vertical projections of osteophytes as a result of the chronic increased erythropoietic activity. Infections, including dental infections, may precipitate a sickle cell crisis; therefore, patients with sickle cell

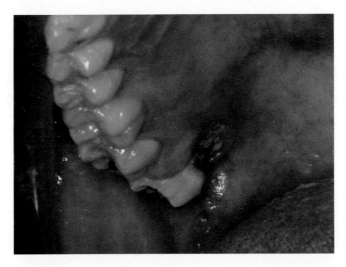

Figure 2.4 Localized soft tissue necrosis secondary to infarcts in a 38-year-old patient with sickle cell disease in sickle cell crisis.

anemia should be assessed dentally on a regular basis, and the importance of good oral hygiene should be emphasized. In patients with poorly controlled disease, there is increased risk of complications from dental procedures secondary to chronic anemia and delayed wound healing, and patients with a history of thrombotic events may be taking anticoagulant medications. If nitrous oxide analgesia is to be administered, high oxygen levels must be maintained.

Thalassemia is another hemoglobinopathy in which Hgb mutations of either the α- or β-globin chains occur, resulting in altered RBC morphology and lysis of these cells. There are a number of variants of this condition, and homozygotes are more severely affected; there are four α-globin genes and two β-globin genes that may be affected. The α-thalassemias are more prevalent in individuals of west African and south Asian descent, while the β-thalassemias are prevalent among individuals of Mediterranean origin. The α-thalassemias are signified by impaired production of the α-globin chain, and presentations range from variable hemolytic anemia (heterozygous) to infant mortality (homozygous). In β-thalassemia, β-globin synthesis is impaired and results in reduced erythropoiesis and hemolysis. In β-thalassemia minor (β-thalassemia trait), affected individuals usually have a mild anemia. β-thalassemia major is associated with severe anemia, systemic dysfunction, and early mortality. Oral manifestations of thalassemia syndromes include dentofacial occlusal abnormalities and iron deposition in enamel and dentin, presenting as red/brown teeth discolorations. Radiographic findings include coarse trabecular patterns, multilocular radiolucencies, and the "hair-on-end" presentation that may exist with sickle cell anemia. As with any patient with chronic anemia, poor healing after dental procedures is a concern due to hypovascularity of tissues.

Glucose-6-phosphate dehydrogenase (G6PD) *deficiency* is a hereditary X-linked enzyme defect that causes episodic hemolysis (abnormal breakdown of red blood cells). The enzyme dysfunction leads to low levels of glutathione, a molecule that when present in normal concentration protects erythrocytes from oxidants. The most commonly affected groups include African-Americans and individuals of Mediterranean origin. Hemolytic episodes occur with the intake of oxidant drugs, such as dapsone or sulfasalazine. Diagnosis can be made through a simple blood test that detects the presence of G6PD, and management requires avoidance of known oxidant drugs.

2.3.2.4.3 *Aplastic anemia*

Aplastic anemia is a hematologic disease that affects the entire hematopoietic system and may be caused by immunosuppressive agents or immune disorders, triggered by medications, or may be idiopathic. As a result of bone marrow failure, there is a depletion of all blood cells (pancytopenia), though RBCs are normochromic and normocytic in appearance. Diagnosis is made by detecting decreased counts of RBCs, WBCs, and platelets, which is then confirmed by bone marrow biopsy demonstrating an acellular marrow. This condition is clinically characterized by pallor, susceptibility to infections, and hemorrhagic diathesis. *Fanconi anemia* is an inherited variant of aplastic anemia that is associated with short stature, learning disability, skeletal and visceral anomalies, and increased risk of cancer, including oropharyngeal squamous cell carcinoma. *Dyskeratosis congenita* is a rare congenital disorder that may present with severe aplastic anemia, and clinical manifestations may include oral and genital leukoplakias that are predisposed for malignant transformation. Infection and bleeding are major concerns in patients with aplastic anemia; therefore, only emergency dental care should be performed until the disease is controlled, and precautions must be taken prior to performing dental procedures (see chapters 3 and 4).

2.3.3 White blood cells

The purpose of the immune system is to identify potentially infectious agents as foreign and to eliminate them from the body. The immune response can be divided into two systems. The innate system represents the first line of defense in which leukocytes (natural killer cells, mast cells, eosinophils, basophils, macrophages, neutrophils, and dendritic cells) fight infection and defend the body via phagocytosis, encapsulating foreign organisms and destroying them. The acquired or adaptive system involves lymphocytes (B-cells and T-cells) that develop a specific response to each infectious agent. The acquired immune response has high specificity for a particular pathogen and also has memory, which enables the body to prevent the same infectious agent from causing disease later.

The predominant cells of the immune system are leukocytes, which originate from hematopoietic stem cells in the bone marrow or lymphoid tissue. *Granulocytes* are leukocytes that have distinctive granules in the cytoplasm and consist of neutrophils, basophils, and eosinophils. Lymphocytes and monocytes make up the *agranulocytes* or *mononuclear leukocytes*. T-lymphocytes are produced in the thymus and create the cell-mediated immune response, while B-lymphocytes from the bone marrow differentiate into plasma cells and memory B-cells to make up the humoral response, mediated by antibody production and secretion.

Reference values of leukocytes are detailed in Alert Box 2.3. *Leukocytosis* is an increase in WBCs and is usually caused by an increase in only one type of leukocyte. Leukocytosis of a temporary nature may occur during acute infection; trauma or tissue injury; acute hemorrhage; use of certain drugs such as corticosteroids, epinephrine, and those used for general anesthesia; or physiologic changes resulting from stress, exercise, temperature changes, nausea, vomiting, and/or seizures. Leukocytosis that is permanent and progressive suggests the possibility of leukemia and requires further work-up. *Leukopenia* is a decrease in normal levels of WBCs and may be idiopathic or may develop secondary to viral infections, medications that cause bone marrow depression, and primary bone marrow disorders such as aplastic anemia and myelodysplastic syndrome (a hematologic condition characterized by ineffective

Alert Box 2.3 WBC Reference ranges and restrictions/modifications for dental treatment.*

Risk level	WBC count (cells/mm³)	Medical consultation recommended?	Interventions
Low (normal)	4–11,000	No	None
Moderate	11,001–30,000 (leukocytosis) 500–3,999 (leukopenia)	Yes	None
High	> 30,000	Yes	High: Obtain medical consultation, may indicate malignancy
	< 500		Low: Consider antibiotic therapy prior to and following invasive dental procedures

*See chapter 4.

production of myeloid blood cells [leukocytes] and risk of transformation to acute myelogenous leukemia). A patient with severe leukopenia is susceptible to oral and systemic infection (see chapter 4). Patients on prolonged steroid therapy may have an impaired leukocyte response, therefore increasing susceptibility to infection (see chapters 4 and 5). The differential white blood cell count is the total count of circulating white blood cells differentiated into the five types of leukocytes, each of which performs a specific function. More information about the functions of leukocytes and the differential counts is addressed in chapter 4.

2.4 Serum chemistry and electrolytes

Blood chemistry and electrolyte testing measures several blood analytes with a single sample of blood, and standard panels have been developed to screen for abnormalities or assess body system function. See Table 2.4 for basic serum chemistry and electrolyte values discussed in this chapter. Shorthand notation for common chemistry values, known as the *Chem 7*, is illustrated in Figure 2.5.

2.4.1 Liver function

The liver serves a primary role of synthesis and breakdown of products for metabolism. Bilirubin is a by-product of normal erythrocyte breakdown and enters the hepatocyte in unconjugated (indirect, not water-soluble) form from portal circulation, after which it is conjugated (direct, conjugated with glucoronic acid, making it water-soluble), transported out of the hepatocyte and prepared for elimination. *Jaundice*, a yellow discoloration most often seen in the skin and sclera of the eyes (Figure 2.6), occurs when bilirubin is retained in the bloodstream and may occur due to increased hemolysis, hepatocyte damage, or destruction of the outflow of bile. In hemolytic anemias, excessive hemolysis results in release of high levels of unconjugated bilirubin in blood. In conditions that cause hepatocyte destruction (e.g., hepatitis, cirrhosis), both unconjugated and conjugated bilirubin

Table 2.4 Reference ranges for serum chemistry, electrolyte, and vitamin/mineral values.

Test	Normal ranges	Clinical significance of values
Serum Chemistry		
Total bilirubin	0.3–1.0 mg/dL	> 1.5 mg/dL: hemolysis or liver dysfunction/blockage
ALT	Males: 10–40 U/L Females: 7–35 U/L	Increase: liver disease If ALT > AST, acute or chronic hepatitis
AST	Males: 14–20 U/L Females: 10–36 U/L	Increase: myocardial infarction, liver disease If AST > ALT (10–100 times normal), active cirrhosis
Alkaline phosphatase	25–100 U/L	Increase: liver disease, bone disease
Albumin	3.5–4.8 g/dL	< 3.0 g/dL: liver disease, acute or chronic inflammatory disease, malnutrition
BUN	6–20 mg/dL	Increase: impaired glomerular function > 50 mg/dL: renal failure
Creatinine	0.6–1.3 mg/dL	Increase: impaired glomerular function > 5 mg/dL: renal failure *Panic value*: 10 mg/dL
Total protein	60–85 mg/dL	Increase: proteinemia, Hodgkin lymphoma, leukemia Decrease: liver disease, acute infection
Electrolytes		
Calcium	8.8–10.4 mg/dL	> 12 mg/dL: hypercalcemia < 4.0 mg/dL: hypocalcemia *Panic values*: > 13 mg/dL: cardiotoxicity, arrhythmias, coma < 3 mg/dL: tetany, convulsions
Potassium	3.5–5.2 mEq/L	*Panic value*: > 6.7 mEq/L: cardiac arrhythmias
Sodium	136–145 mEq/L	< 125 mEq/L: weakness, dehydration > 160 mEq/L: heart failure
Chloride	96–106 mEq/L	< 70 mEq/L: metabolic alkalosis > 120 mEq/L: metabolic acidosis
Vitamins/Minerals		
Iron	Males: 65–175 µg/dL Females: 50–170 µg/dL	< 40 µg/dL: iron deficiency
Ferritin	Males: 20–250 ng/mL Females: 10–120 ng/mL	< 10 ng/mL: iron deficiency
Vitamin B_{12}	200–835 pg/mL	< 100 pg/mL: B_{12} deficiency
Folic acid	2–20 ng/mL	< 1.5 ng/mL: folic acid deficiency
Homocysteine	Males: 4.3–11.4 µmol/L Females: 3.3–10.4 µmol/L	< 6.3 µmol/L: therapeutic target for B_{12} deficiency > 13 µmol/L: B_{12} deficiency, risk factor for cardiovascular disease
Methylmalonic acid	0.08–0.36 µmol/L	> 0.4 µmol/L: B_{12} deficiency

ALT = alanine anminotransferase.
AST = aspartate transaminase.

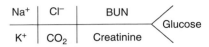

Figure 2.5 Shorthand notation for common chemistry values (Chem 7).

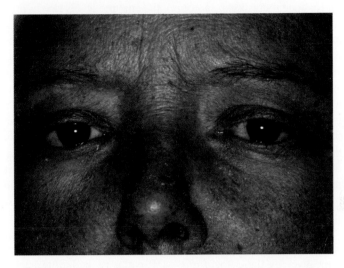

Figure 2.6 Jaundice in the sclera of the eyes affecting a 65-year-old patient with acute hepatitis A.

accumulate. Biliary obstruction will cause an elevated level of conjugated bilirubin in the serum and accumulation in urine.

Coagulopathy (dysfunction affecting the blood's ability to coagulate) occurs in all diseases with hepatocyte damage due to impaired production of coagulation factors and inhibitors. Further, the liver synthesizes five critical vitamin K–dependent clotting factors and fibrinogen (see chapter 3), and since vitamin K is stored in the liver, deficiency of this vitamin can occur with loss of storage sites caused by hepatocellular disease or biliary tract obstruction. Hepatocyte destruction may also lead to portal hypertension and ascites (peritoneal cavity fluid) due to vasculature leaks. In addition, patients with advanced liver disease may experience thrombocytopenia (decreased number of platelets) due to hypersplenism (caused by portal hypertension), resulting in platelet sequestration, and qualitative platelet dysfunction can occur secondary to impaired protein synthesis, causing activation of the fibrinolytic pathway and impaired release of fibrinolytic system inhibitors. Patients with end-stage liver disease are candidates for hepatic transplantation.

Diagnosis of liver dysfunction can be determined by assessing bilirubin levels and liver function tests that measure enzymes that provide information about liver impairment. If total bilirubin levels are elevated, tests of unconjugated and conjugated bilirubin can determine the etiology. Alanine aminotransferase (ALT) is an enzyme found in high concentrations in the liver. Increased serum ALT is a sensitive indicator of liver disease. Aspartate transaminase (AST) is an enzyme present in tissues of high metabolic activity and is released into the circulation following the injury or death of cells. The ALT is more specific than AST for liver disease, but the AST is more sensitive to alcoholic liver disease (cirrhosis). In severe cirrhosis where most of the liver has become functionally fibrotic, the AST and ALT may be normal due to a lack of viable hepatocytes. In these circumstances, other screening algorithms, such as the Child-Pugh score, may be utilized to assess prognosis of chronic end-stage liver disease.

Alkaline phosphatase (ALP) is used as an index of liver and bone disease when correlated with other clinical findings. In liver disease, the blood level of ALP rises when excretion of this enzyme is impaired as a result of obstruction in the biliary tract. In bone disease (e.g., Paget disease, bone metastases, sarcoma), the enzyme levels rise in proportion to new bone cell production resulting from osteoblastic activity and the deposit of calcium in the bones. Albumin is synthesized in the liver and is part of a complex buffer system. Decreased albumin levels are associated with acute and chronic inflammation and infections, particularly liver cirrhosis, renal disease with proteinuria, and gastrointestinal tract leaks. Serum total protein represents the total amount of protein in serum and is made up of albumin and globulin, and low values usually reflect low albumin concentration.

Clinical signs and symptoms of liver disease include the presence of clinical jaundice, affecting the skin, sclera of eyes, and sometimes oral mucosa, as well as gastrointestinal symptoms such as nausea, vomiting, and right upper quadrant pain. When patients with hepatobiliary disease are seen in the dental setting, coagulopathy is a significant concern secondary to inability to synthesize prothrombin and other clotting factors. In patients with chronic hepatitis and all forms of cirrhosis, clotting ability should be assessed prior to performing dentoalveolar surgery, and in patients with advanced liver disease, platelet count should also be evaluated (see chapter 3). For control of post-operative pain, drugs that inhibit platelet adhesion (e.g., NSAIDs) should be avoided. Further, since numerous drugs are metabolized in the liver by the cytochrome p450 pathway, including acetaminophen and opioids, doses should be altered appropriately. Finally, hepatitis B and C viruses are transmissible from actively infected patients and carriers in the dental office environment, underscoring the utmost importance of universal infection control precautions. Post–liver transplant patients may be taking immunosuppressive medications that require further management in the dental setting (see chapter 4).

2.4.2 Kidney function

The kidneys serve numerous important roles, including regulating acid-base and fluid-electrolyte balances of the body, excreting metabolic waste products, and secreting renin, vitamin D, and erythropoietin, which regulate blood pressure, calcium metabolism, and production of erythrocytes, respectively. With kidney dysfunction, nephrons are destroyed and glomerular filtration becomes diminished, resulting in loss of fluid-electrolyte and acid-base balance and decreased ability to concentrate the urine. Eventually, the glomerular vessels become narrowed (microangiopathy), which triggers the release of renin, and through the renin-angiotensin system, leads to vasoconstriction and hypertension. As vessel walls thicken, the filtration of waste substances and ion exchange mechanisms becomes impaired, with both retention of waste products (uremia) and loss of proteins (proteinuria), presenting clinically as polyuria and nocturia. Acid-base imbalance causes metabolic acidosis (from diminished ability to excrete hydrogen ions) and hyperkalemia (increased potassium), which at high levels can cause fatal cardiac dysrhythmias. Decreased erythropoietin production leads to anemia, and the inability of the kidneys to convert vitamin D into its active form causes hypocalcemia (resulting in calcium transport out of bone) and secondary hyperparathyroidism (which may result in renal osteodystrophy). Renal dysfunction is progressive and results in end-stage renal disease (ESRD), whereby patients must undergo hemodialysis or renal transplantation.

The following tests are useful in assessing kidney function and are obtained through a basic metabolic panel: blood urea nitrogen (BUN), creatinine, glucose (see chapter 5), and the electrolytes sodium, chloride, carbon dioxide, potassium, phosphate, and calcium. Elevated creatinine and BUN levels measure uremia and correspond to the degree of kidney dysfunction. BUN measures the nitrogen portion of urea and is used as an index of glomerular function in the production and excretion of urine. Kidney function impairment and rapid protein catabolism will result in an elevated BUN level. A significantly increased BUN is conclusive evidence of severely impaired glomerular function. Creatinine is a by-product in the breakdown of muscle creatine phosphate resulting from energy metabolism. It is produced at a constant rate and is removed from the body by the kidneys. A disorder of kidney function reduces excretion of creatinine, resulting in increased blood creatinine levels. Thus, creatinine levels provide a proxy measure of the glomerular filtration rate. Creatinine is a very sensitive indicator of kidney disease, especially early dysfunction.

In patients with renal dysfunction, medications that are excreted in the kidneys should be dose-altered to the level of renal function. For the ESRD patient on dialysis (typical dialysis regimen is 3 days/week), dental treatment should be performed on non-dialysis days due to heparinization during dialysis, mechanical destruction of platelets, and patient fatigue after dialysis treatment. ESRD patients are at risk for excessive bleeding and infection, so precautions should be addressed prior to dental treatment (see chapters 3 and 4). Post–kidney transplant patients may be taking immunosuppressive medications that require further management in the dental setting (see chapter 4).

Oral manifestations of renal disease typically occur at late stages. *Uremic stomatitis* may occur in ESRD patients with severe uremia as a result of ammonia being present in the saliva. Clinically, oral lesions consist of mucosal tissues with a gray pseudomembrane or ulcerations and a complaint of dysgeusia. *Renal osteodystrophy* as a consequence of secondary hyperparathyroidism (Figure 2.7; section 2.4.3) may present as loss of lamina dura around teeth, ground-glass trabecular pattern, and brown tumors, which are lesions that are composed of multinucleated giant cells, hemosiderin, and fibroblasts and clinically appear brown.

2.4.3   *Electrolytes*

Electrolytes are critical for cellular function and homeostasis (Table 2.4). Typically, the concentration of cations (i.e., Na+, K+, Ca++, Mg+) is higher in the plasma, while anions (Cl-, HPO4-) tend to be higher in the interstitial fluid. Electrolyte values are useful in assessing acid-base balance.

The concentration of total calcium in the blood reflects parathyroid function, calcium metabolism, and malignancy activity. Hyperparathyroidism and cancer that invades bone are the most common causes of hypercalcemia. Parathyroid hormone controls calcium levels by influencing bone resorption and is feedback-regulated by serum calcium. Primary hyperparathyroidism is caused by benign tumors (adenomas) or parathyroid gland hyperplasia, while secondary hyperparathyroidism usually reflects renal disease with parathyroid hyperactivity to maintain adequate serum calcium levels. Classic signs and symptoms of hypercalcemia and hyperparathyroidism are summarized by the mnemonic "stones, bones, abdominal groans, and psychiatric moans" and may include nephrocalcinosis (kidney stones), bone pain and sometimes pathologic fractures due to elevated parathyroid activity (bones), constipation, nausea and vomiting (abdominal groans), and fatigue, confusion, and

(a)

(b)

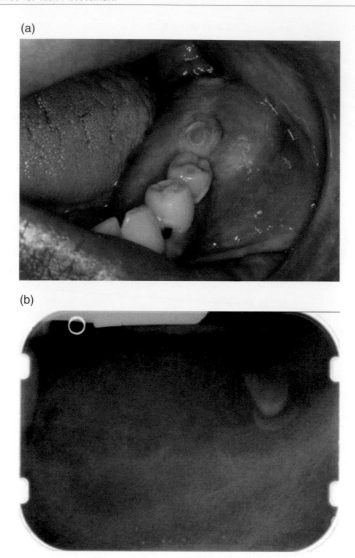

Figure 2.7   Clinical (a) and radiographic (b) presentation of renal osteodystrophy in a patient with end-stage renal disease. Note the radiographic ground-glass trabecular pattern of bone.

depression (psychiatric moans). The dental findings for primary and secondary hyperparathyroidism are indistinguishable.

Potassium is the primary buffer within the cell and helps to maintain osmotic pressure. Along with calcium, potassium controls heart contraction and cardiac output. Potassium and sodium are important in the renal regulation of acid-base balance, as hydrogen ions are substituted for sodium and potassium ions in the renal tubule. Increased potassium levels (hyperkalemia) occur when K+ shifts from cells to intracellular fluid with inadequate renal excretion and can contribute to metabolic acidosis and cardiac arrhythmias.

Sodium and chloride function to maintain osmotic pressure and acid-base balance. Alteration of sodium chloride level causes changes in water balance and may be related to hydration, renal, and/or cardiovascular health. These alterations are seldom a primary problem, but they are important in the correction of hypokalemic alkalosis.

2.5   Suggested literature

Chobanian AV, Bakris GL, Black HR, et al. Seventh Report of the Joint National Committee on Prevention, Detection, Evaluation, and Treatment of High Blood Pressure. Hypertension 2003;42(6):1206–1252.

Da Fonseca M, Oueis HS, Casamassimo PS. Sickle cell anemia: A review for the pediatric dentist. Pediatr Dent 2007;29(2):159–169.

Fauci AS, Braunwald E, Kasper DL, Hauser SL, Longo DL, Jameson JL, Loscaizo J, eds. Harrison's Principles of Internal Medicine, 17th ed. http://www.accessmedicine.com.

Firriolo FJ. Dental management of patients with end-stage liver disease. Dent Clin North Am 2006;50(4): 563–590.

Fischbach F, Dunning MB. A Manual of Laboratory and Diagnostic Tests, 8th ed. Philadelphia: Lippincott, Williams & Wilkins, 2008.

FitzSimons D, Francois G, De Carli G, et al. Hepatitis B virus, hepatitis C virus and other blood-borne infections in healthcare workers: Guidelines for prevention and management in industrialised countries. Occup Environ Med 2008;65(7):446–451.

Koeppen BM. The kidney and acid-base regulation. Adv Physiol Educ 2009;33(4):275–281.

Raja K, Coletti DP. Management of the dental patient with renal disease. Dent Clin North Am 2006;50(4): 529–545.

3 Potential for Bleeding

3.0 INTRODUCTION

Dental patients may be at risk for abnormal peri- and post-operative bleeding due to a variety of inherited and acquired conditions that affect normal hemostasis. First and foremost in assessing this risk is obtaining a comprehensive medical and medication history, and patients should be specifically asked if they have bleeding or healing problems: *Do you bleed or bruise easily? Do you have trouble with prolonged bleeding if you accidentally cut yourself? Do you have trouble with frequent nosebleeds?* In patients who are considered to be at risk, appropriate ordering and interpretation of laboratory tests is warranted in most cases to evaluate the potential for bleeding complications. In some situations, abnormal or prolonged bleeding following a dental surgical procedure may be the initial presentation of an underlying bleeding disorder.

Hemostasis can be divided into four phases: (1) vascular, (2) platelet aggregation, (3) coagulation cascade, and (4) fibrinolysis. Following tissue injury, localized vasoconstriction minimizes blood loss. Exposure of the damaged vasculature activates platelets, which aggregate and rapidly form a temporary platelet plug. These early steps initiate the coagulation cascade, leading to fibrin formation that strengthens the initial clot. This is followed by fibrinolysis, in which the clot is degraded proteolytically, a necessary step for normal healing. Primary hemostasis is mediated primarily by adequate numbers of functioning platelets and occurs within minutes. Secondary hemostasis depends on normal levels of coagulation factors and takes place over hours to days. Rarely, underlying disorders in collagen and vessel wall integrity can result in clinically significant bleeding. These include metabolic and vitamin deficiencies (e.g., scurvy), collagen vascular disorders (e.g., Ehlers-Danlos syndrome, hereditary hemorrhagic telangiectasia), and endocrine disorders (e.g., Cushing syndrome). The majority of bleeding disorders are due to quantitative and qualitative abnormalities with platelets or coagulation proteins. Depending on the specific diagnosis and severity of abnormalities, bleeding can generally be anticipated prior to performing dental procedures, and measures must be taken to minimize risk of excess blood loss and the need for post-operative emergency management.

Risk Assessment and Oral Diagnostics in Clinical Dentistry, First Edition.
Dena J. Fischer, Nathaniel S. Treister and Andres Pinto.
© 2013 John Wiley & Sons, Inc. Published 2013 by John Wiley & Sons, Inc.

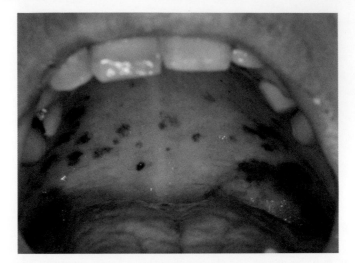

Figure 3.1 Multiple palatal petechiae and ecchymoses in a patient with severe thrombocytopenia secondary to aplastic anemia.

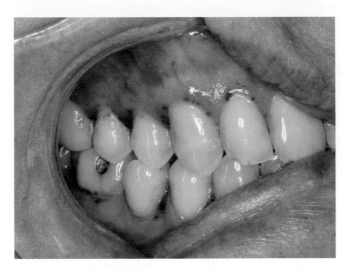

Figure 3.2 Petechiae of the marginal gingiva in a patient with severe thrombocytopenia secondary to acute leukemia.

Oral soft tissue lesions, including petechiae (small red extravasation lesions), ecchymoses (larger extravasation lesions), and hematomas (exophytic rubbery lesions composed of clotted blood), are frequently encountered in patients with clinically significant bleeding disorders (Figures 3.1–3.4). The tongue, buccal mucosa, and soft palate are commonly affected due to normal functional tissue contact. These lesions are usually painless and asymptomatic, and all lesions, even large hematomas, will resolve spontaneously with correction of the underlying abnormality. Of note, all of the above lesions can develop secondary to trauma even in the absence of an underlying bleeding disorder, although they are not observed at nearly the same frequency.

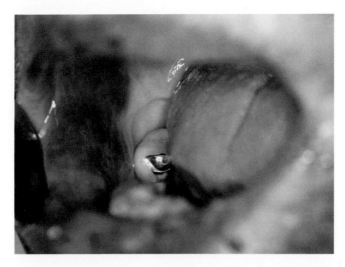

Figure 3.3   Diffuse ecchymosis of the right buccal mucosa in an anticoagulated patient following an accidental fall.

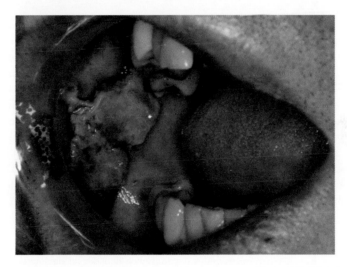

Figure 3.4   Exophytic hematoma of the right buccal mucosa in a patient with severe thrombocytopenia associated with advanced multiple myeloma.

Dental procedures that involve any type of soft or hard tissue damage can potentially cause bleeding. The highest-risk procedures include dentoalveolar surgery, in particular multiple extractions, periodontal surgical procedures, including deep scaling and root planing, and soft tissue biopsies (Figure 3.5). Lower risk procedures in which excessive bleeding is rarely encountered include rubber dam clamp placement, use of retraction cord and local anesthesia injections. However, in patients with severe coagulopathies, even a simple inferior alveolar nerve block can induce life-threatening hematoma formation. Specific considerations are highlighted in this chapter.

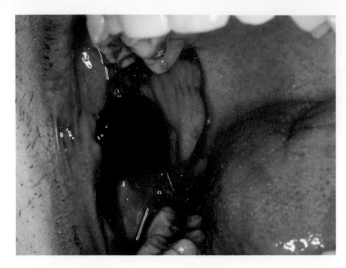

Figure 3.5 Persistent bleeding following a punch biopsy in a patient with previously undiagnosed Factor XI deficiency.

3.1 Platelets

Platelets are generated from megakaryocytes in the bone marrow, circulate in the blood, and become activated when they come into contact with an injured blood vessel. An adequate number of circulating functional platelets are critical for primary hemostasis. In addition to exposure to the damaged vessel matrix, platelets also require the presence of von Willebrand factor (vWF), a plasma protein that facilitates initial platelet adhesion and stabilizes Factor VIII (FVIII; section 3.2.2.2.2). Following adhesion, platelets degranulate and release a number of intracellular components, including the potent nucleotide adenosine diphosphate (ADP), that recruit additional platelets, mediate aggregation, and initiate coagulation. Patients who are profoundly thrombocytopenic (less than 20,000 cells/mm^3; Alert Box 3.1) are at significant risk for spontaneous bleeding and are often supported with platelet transfusions to maintain a minimal level of 20,000 cells/mm^3.

Alert Box 3.1 Platelet count values and restrictions/modifications for dental treatment.*

Risk level	Platelet count (cells/mm^3)	Medical consultation recommended?	Interventions
Low	>100,000	No	None
Moderate	50,000–100,000	Yes	Consider localized measures
High	20,000–50,000	Yes	Localized measures indicated, consider platelet transfusion
Panic	<20,000	Yes	Requires platelet transfusion

*For procedures in which bleeding is anticipated.

3.1.1   *Platelet tests*

The most important test of primary hemostasis is the platelet count. Any patient suspected of having a decreased number of circulating platelets should have a platelet count obtained prior to any invasive surgical procedures. Several platelet function tests are available, but these are not widely used and should generally be ordered by a consulting hematologist when indicated.

3.1.1.1   *Platelet count*
Normal platelet counts range from 150,000 to 450,000 cells/mm^3 (Alert Box 3.1). While there is large variation among the population, an individual's count tends to remain within a certain range. The platelet count is purely quantitative and does not measure platelet functionality.

3.1.1.2   *Bleeding time*
The bleeding time is a fairly crude test of platelet function in which the skin is incised and observed for primary hemostasis in a standardized manner. This test is a poor indicator of mucosal and oral surgery induced bleeding and is therefore of limited clinical utility in dentistry.

3.1.1.3   *Liver function tests*
Since patients with advanced liver disease may present with both quantitative and qualitative platelet disorders in addition to clotting defects, liver function tests may provide additional information regarding an individual patient's risk of bleeding (see chapter 2). Ordering of liver function tests for evaluation of primary hemostasis should be driven by patient history. The utilization of these tests for evaluation of secondary hemostasis is discussed below (section 3.2.2.2.3).

3.1.2   *Platelet abnormalities*

Conditions that lead to a decreased number of platelets, called *thrombocytopenia*, or dysfunctional platelet activity can cause abnormal bleeding. Thrombocytopenia may be due to decreased production, increased splenic sequestration, or accelerated destruction of platelets, while etiologies of dysfunctional platelet activity include medications, von Willebrand disease (vWD), and hematologic malignancies. These patients may present with gingival bleeding, excessive perioperative bleeding, or persistent post-operative bleeding due to insufficient primary hemostasis. Management is highly dependent on the nature and severity of the underlying condition as well as the planned procedure for which bleeding is anticipated.

3.1.2.1   *Medication-induced*
Certain medications have antiplatelet activity and are used therapeutically for management and prevention of thromboembolic disease (Table 3.1). However, many patients also take these medications for other reasons and may be unaware of their increased risk for bleeding. Risk assessment requires a careful medication history including reason for taking the medication, an understanding of the different mechanisms of action of the various antiplatelet medications, and use and interpretation of appropriate laboratory tests when indicated.

Table 3.1 Medications administered in the outpatient setting that may increase the risk of oral bleeding.

Therapeutic indication	Medication class	Examples	Mechanism	Dose modifications?	Recommended diagnostic test(s)	Implications for dental care
Antithrombotic	Salicylates	Acetasylic acid	Irreversibly inhibits prostaglandin synthesis	None	None	Potential delay in *primary* hemostasis
	NSAIDs	Ibuprofen	Reversibly inhibits prostaglandin synthesis	None	None	Anticipate *early* oozing/bleeding
	Platelet aggregation inhibitors	Clopiogrel Prasugrel Ticlopidine	Inhibits ADP-induced platelet aggregation	None	None	Local measures only
		Dipyridamole	Inhibits thromboxane synthase, inhibits cellular reuptake of adenosine, inhibits adenosine deaminase and phosphodiesterase		None	
		Cilostazol	Inhibits cellular phosphodiesterase		None	
	Antiplatelet agents	Anagrelide	Reduces platelet count through inhibition of cyclic AMP and phosphodiesterase III	None	None	
Anticoagulant	Low-molecular weight heparins	Enoxaparin Dalteparin Tinzaparin	Binds to and increases activity of antithrombin III, inhibiting thrombin and Factor Xa	None	None	Potential delay in *secondary* hemostasis
	Coumarins	Warfarin	Inhibits vitamin K–dependent coagulation factor synthesis (II, VII, IX, X, proteins C and S)	None	PT/INR	Anticipate *late* oozing/bleeding
	Direct thrombin inhibitors	Dabigatran etexilate	Inhibits thrombin, blocks fibrin formation	None	None	Local measures only
	Factor Xa inhibitors	Rivaroxaban	Blocks active site of factor Xa	None	None	

3.1.2.1.1   *Acetasylic acid and non-steroidal anti-inflammatory agents*
Acetasylic acid (ASA) is one of the most commonly prescribed medications used for thromboembolic prophylaxis and is also taken routinely for its analgesic properties. ASA inhibits prostaglandin synthetase, which blocks cyclooxygenase activity, resulting in decreased production of prostaglandins and thromboxanes, both of which are required for platelet function. This effect is irreversible and lasts 7–10 days, the lifetime of a platelet. Most of the nonsteroidal anti-inflammatory agents (NSAIDs) have a similar but reversible effect, with complete restoration of platelet function within 3 days of medication discontinuation. NSAIDs that specifically inhibit cyclooxygenase 2 (COX2 inhibitors, e.g., celecoxib) rather than cyclooxygenase 1 (COX1, e.g., ibuprofen, naproxen) have minimal impact on platelet aggregation and bleeding risk.

3.1.2.1.2   *ADP inhibitors*
Clopidogrel bisulfate (Plavix) inhibits platelet aggregation by blocking ADP and is increasingly being used, often long term, for prevention of thromboembolic disease or prophylaxis following coronary artery stent placement. Prasurgel (Effient) is another ADP inhibitor that is Food and Drug Administration (FDA) approved for use in patients with acute coronary syndrome. Since the number of circulating platelets is not affected, the platelet count is not a useful test in patients taking these medications. Numerous studies have demonstrated that in almost all cases, dental surgical procedures, including multiple extractions, can be safely performed using basic localized hemostatic measures (section 3.2.3).

3.1.2.1.3   *Chemotherapy agents*
Cytoreductive chemotherapy agents often cause bone marrow suppression and a subsequent decrease in white blood cells, as well as platelets, due to destruction of rapidly dividing hematopoietic stem cells. The platelet count typically drops 6–10 days after initiation of therapy and restores gradually over a 1- to 2-week period after completion of therapy. Some agents and specific regimens are more likely to cause significant thrombocytopenia than others. Patients on multiple cycles of chemotherapy may be thrombocytopenic for extended periods with only very short periods of full count recovery.

3.1.2.1.4   *Other medications*
A number of other medications, including over-the-counter and herbal preparations, have been reported to be associated with bleeding. Selective serotonin reuptake inhibitors (SSRIs), such as citalopram and fluoxetine, can potentially inhibit platelet aggregation. In some cases, especially when SSRIs are taken in combination with other antiplatelet or anticoagulatory agents, or when there is a history of an underlying bleeding disorder or coagulopathy, increased bleeding may occur. It remains controversial whether any over-the-counter herbal agents, such as ginkgo biloba, garlic, St. John's wort, and saw palmetto, truly inhibit platelet function, resulting in clinically significant bleeding. Alcohol can block platelet aggregation and activation, decrease levels of coagulation factors, and increase fibrinolysis. When consumed moderately, this is believed to be the reason for the cardioprotective properties of alcohol, but clinically significant bleeding is rare except in cases of cirrhosis due to complications of liver dysfunction (see chapter 2).

3.1.2.2   *Congenital*
Congenital platelet disorders are rare and include *Glanzmann thrombasthenia* and *platelet-type von Willebrand disease*. Glanzmann thrombasthenia is characterized by a

(a)

(b)

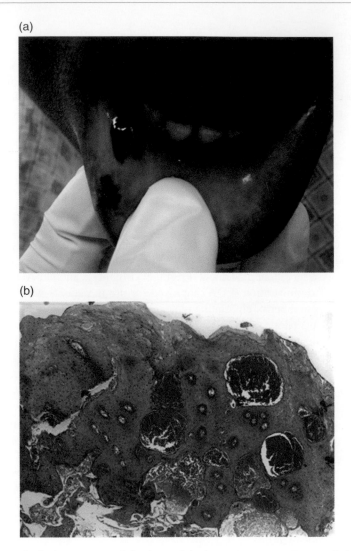

Figure 3.6 Multiple hematomas of the lower labial mucosa in a patient with lupus-associated thrombocytopenia (a). The histopathology in (b) demonstrates sub- and intraepithelial collections of extravasated blood.

functional defect in the platelet membrane glycoproteins IIb and IIIa, leading to increased bleeding due to decreased aggregation. Platelet-type vWD presents clinically as a primary platelet disorder compared with the more common forms of vWD that are more coagulopathic in nature and are associated with more significant bleeding.

3.1.2.3 *Acquired*
There are several acquired platelet disorders that may present as isolated conditions or as a component of a hematologic disease. Immune thrombocytopenic purpura (ITP, also known as idiopathic thrombocytopenic purpura) is a generally indolent disease that is most commonly seen in female young adults, characterized by antibody-mediated platelet destruction. ITP can be associated with systemic diseases, such as can be seen in systemic lupus

erythematosus (Figure 3.6). Clinical features include petechiae and purpura of the skin and oral cavity as well as more serious internal mucosal bleeding. Long-term immunosuppressive therapy is the mainstay of management for ITP.

Thrombotic thrombocytopenia purpura (TTP) is a serious acute disorder that may occur in association with malignancy, pregnancy, or high-dose chemotherapy. Clinical features include thrombocytopenia, microangiopathic hemolytic anemia, neurologic abnormalities, and renal dysfunction. Despite intensive inpatient management, TTP may result in death.

Thrombocytopenia can be an important component of bone marrow disorders including myelodysplastic syndrome, aplastic anemia, and leukemia. In these conditions, the bone marrow simply does not produce sufficient numbers of megakaryocytes, resulting in a reduced number of circulating platelets. In some cases there is also a degree of platelet dysfunction.

Patients with end-stage renal disease (see chapter 2) and uremia may develop dysfunctional platelet activity due to a defect in the glycoprotein IIb-IIIa complex. Since this is a qualitative platelet defect secondary to uremic toxins that decrease platelet adhesiveness, the number of platelets is unaffected.

3.2   Coagulation

Coagulation encompasses all of the carefully coordinated steps of secondary hemostasis, in which the initial platelet plug is further reinforced by the deposition of fibrin, making the clot stronger and more resistant to fibrinolysis by plasmin. Many of the proteins involved in coagulation are synthesized in the liver and are dependent on the presence of vitamin K. The coagulation cascade is composed of intrinsic and extrinsic pathways, both of which include a series of bioamplification steps that meet at the common pathway. The intrinsic pathway is initiated by activation of Factor XII by surface contact with exposed endothelial tissue. The extrinsic pathway does not require tissue contact for activation but rather is dependent on the release of thromboplastin, or tissue factor, that binds to Factor VII. The thromboplastin/Factor VII complex is capable of activating Factors IX (FIX) and X, linking the extrinsic and intrinsic pathways and initiating activation of the common pathway.

In the common pathway, prothrombin is converted to thrombin, which subsequently converts circulating, insoluble fibrinogen to fibrin. The polymerization of fibrin creates a gel-like substance that stabilizes the primary platelet plug. Factor XIII, also activated by thrombin, cross-links the fibrin molecules, further strengthening the clot. Since this is a carefully controlled and regulated system, fibrinolysis is initiated at the same time as the coagulation process, thereby allowing for normal wound remodeling and healing. Ultimately, plasminogen is converted to plasmin (mediated in large part by tissue plasminogen activator [tPA]), which then degrades fibrinogen and fibrin into fibrin degradation products.

3.2.1   *Tests of coagulation*

Laboratory testing of coagulation values is the primary way in which risk of bleeding due to coagulopathy is evaluated. The partial thromboplastin time (PTT) measures the intrinsic and common pathways, while the prothrombin time (PT) measures the extrinsic and common pathways (Alert Box 3.2).

Alert Box 3.2 Coagulation test values and restrictions/modifications for dental treatment.

Risk level	aPTT	INR	Interventions
Low (normal)		0.8–1.0	None
Moderate	21–35 seconds	1.0–3.5	Consider localized measures
High	>35 seconds	≥3.5	Localized measures indicated
			In cases of severe coagulopathy, may require FFP or specific factor replacement, depending on underlying etiology

3.2.1.1 *aPTT*

The activated partial thromboplastin time (aPTT), more commonly referred to as the PTT, measures the efficacy of the intrinsic and common coagulation pathways. It is useful in hospital settings to monitor treatment effects of heparin therapy. However, PTT is not beneficial in patients taking low-molecular-weight heparin therapy (section 3.2.2.1). PTT is also used to assess bleeding risk in hemophiliacs, as this test includes Factors VIII and IX (section 3.2.2.2.1).

3.2.1.2 *PT/INR*

The PT measures Factors II, V, VII, X, and fibrinogen of the extrinsic coagulation pathway. It is reported as the International Normalized Ratio (INR), which standardizes PT results across labs that might differ due to various reagents. The INR is elevated in patients taking oral anticoagulant therapy and with advanced liver disease. A normal INR range is 0.8–1.2, and depending on the specific clinical indication for anticoagulation, patients on anticoagulation therapy are generally maintained between 2.0 and 3.0. Patients on short-term prophylaxis for deep vein thrombosis (DVT) are maintained between 2.0 and 2.5; the majority of indications, including treatment and long-term prophylaxis for DVT, atrial fibrillation, and post–myocardial infarction are maintained between 2.0 and 3.0; and patients with recurrent DVT and prosthetic heart valves may be maintained at levels up to 3.5. An elevated INR (1.5 or greater) in a non-anticoagulated patient should raise the suspicion of underlying liver disease.

3.2.2 Coagulation abnormalities

In theory, any deficiency in the coagulation cascade has the potential to result in prolonged bleeding. While there are many well-characterized inherited coagulation disorders, the most commonly affected components associated with clinically significant bleeding include vWF, FVIII, and FIX. However, the most common cause of prolonged coagulation is iatrogenic pharmacologic anticoagulation for the prevention of thromboembolic disease. Patients with abnormalities in coagulation tend to demonstrate ecchymoses (Figure 3.3), rather than smaller petechiae seen with thrombocytopenia, and delayed bleeding with initially normal clotting following injury or surgical procedures. Ultimately, similar to patients with platelet abnormalities, management is highly dependent on the nature and severity of the underlying condition as well as the planned procedure for which bleeding is anticipated.

3.2.2.1 *Anticoagulant drugs*

Heparin is a potent and fast-acting anticoagulant that binds antithrombin III, which inhibits several coagulation factors, resulting in the inhibition of fibrin formation. Heparin works quickly and is therefore ideal for prophylaxis of thromboembolic disease in hospitalized patients undergoing surgery and those restricted to bed rest. Heparin is administered either intravenously or subcutaneously. Protamine sulfate rapidly reverses heparin's anticoagulant effects. Low-molecular-weight heparins (LMWHs), such as enoxaparin (Lovenox, Clexane), ardeparin (Normiflo), and dalteparin (Fragmin), are adminstered subcutaneously once or twice a day and are rarely associated with clinically significant bleeding. LMWHs permit outpatient treatment of thromboembolic conditions that previously required inpatient hospitalization for unfractionated heparin administration. After careful coordination with a patient's cardiologist, individuals may undergo oral/dental surgical procedures in an outpatient setting after LMWH administration.

Coumarin anticoagulants include warfarin and dicumarol (Coumadin, Bristol-Myers Squibb, Princeton, NJ) and are taken orally for the prophylaxis and/or treatment of thromboembolic disease and thromboembolic complications associated with atrial fibrillation and/or cardiac valve replacement. Coumarin anticoagulants block vitamin K activity, thereby reducing levels of vitamin K–dependent coagulation factors and limiting thrombin production. Compared with heparin, the duration of action is much longer, taking several days to reach full activity. Furthermore, fluctuation in levels can occur, necessitating routine long-term monitoring of anticoagulation by the INR (section 3.2.1.2). Drug interactions can increase (e.g., metronidazole, penicillin, erythromycin, cephalosporins, tetracycline, fluconazole) or decrease (e.g., barbiturates, ascorbic acid, dicloxacillin) coumarin potency, as demonstrated by changes in the INR. The anticoagulant effect can be rapidly reversed by infusion of fresh frozen plasma, or more gradually by treatment with vitamin K.

Dabigatran etexilate (Pradaxa) is a recently FDA-approved direct inhibitor of thrombin indicated for prophylaxis of thromboembolism and stroke in patients with atrial fibrillation. Monitoring of anticoagulation by INR is not required for this agent.

3.2.2.2 *Coagulopathic conditions*
A number of inherited and acquired coagulopathic disorders can cause bleeding. Depending on the factor(s) affected and the levels of functional factor(s), bleeding can range from mild to severe. Management is primarily driven by the specific disorder, an individual patient's history of bleeding, and bleeding-related complications.

3.2.2.2.1 *Hemophilias*
Hemophilia A and B are X-linked recessive bleeding disorders seen almost exclusively in males, although female carriers may demonstrate mild phenotypes. Hemophilia A is characterized by deficiency of FVIII, whereas hemophilia B is defined as a deficiency of FIX; both are associated with varying degrees of bleeding depending on the severity of disease. Significant clinical bleeding is not seen unless factor levels are less than 1% of normal. Bleeding tends to be deep in the body, resulting in a multitude of complications, the most significant including hemarthroses, gastrointestinal bleeding, and intracranial bleeding. Severe cases require continuous prophylactic factor replacement therapy; however, development of inhibitors (blocking antibodies) against the replacement coagulation factors is a serious complication.

Management of bleeding in hemophiliacs, including prophylaxis in anticipation of an oral surgical procedure or even a local anesthetic injection that may damage a blood vessel, requires factor replacement and must be coordinated by the patient's hematologist. The dose and duration of factor replacement treatment are determined by the nature of the procedure as well as the patient's individual history. Development of inhibiting antibodies is a serious complication that can significantly impact management. The development of inhibitors occurs as the body recognizes the replacement factor as "foreign," rendering the replacement factor ineffective. This complication can be managed by increasing factor replacement levels or administering other factor replacement in an attempt to "bypass" the inhibitors. Desmopressin acetate (DDAVP), which can be delivered intranasally, increases circulating FVIII levels and can be effective in less severe cases, eliminating the need for factor replacement. In emergency situations, fresh frozen plasma (FFP) can be infused as it contains both FVIII and FIX.

3.2.2.2.2   *von Willebrand disease*

vWF is a multimeric protein that is involved in platelet adhesion and also acts as a carrier for FVIII. vWD can be due to low levels or functional and/or structural deficiencies in vWF, resulting in a wide range of clinical bleeding. It is the most common inherited bleeding disorder, and in its most common form, Type 1, clinical manifestations are generally mild, although severe bleeding is possible. Type 1 is characterized by decreased levels of vWF and accompanying lower FVIII levels, Type 2 by qualitative/functional changes, and Type 3 by absence of vWF and very low levels of FVIII. Management is determined by the type and severity of vWD. DDAVP is generally sufficient for most Type 1 patients; however, more severe cases may require FVIII replacement therapy or platelet transfusions.

3.2.2.2.3   *Liver disease*

Patients with hepatic disease (e.g., chronic hepatitis, cirrhosis, hepatocellular carcinoma) may not have sufficient synthesis of necessary coagulation factors, placing them at potentially high risk for bleeding. In advanced liver disease, thrombocytopenia can also be encountered. Since vitamin K is stored in the liver, patients with advanced disease also have decreased production of vitamin K–dependent clotting factors and fibrinogen. Liver disease is monitored primarily by blood tests (see chapter 2), and values that are elevated may indicate disease activity and organ dysfunction. Due to the widespread deficiency in coagulation factors, coagulation tests should be monitored in patients with advanced liver disease, and FFP may be required for bleeding prophylaxis or management.

3.2.3   Guidelines for dental treatment

3.2.3.1   *General considerations*

Patients at risk for bleeding must be carefully evaluated prior to oral procedures that are likely to result in any degree of bleeding. These include deep scaling and root planing, periodontal surgeries, extractions and other surgical procedures including implant placement, and in the case of hemophilias, even local anesthesia injections. Endodontic therapy that does not extend significantly beyond the apex does not cause significant bleeding and can be safely performed in patients at risk for bleeding. Pertinent laboratory values should be obtained within 24 hours of the procedure. Depending on the underlying disorder and its severity, measures may have to be taken prior to, during, and following oral surgical procedures (Table 3.2). Consultation with a hematologist or cardiologist is recommended in more complicated cases, and in some situations treatment may be best provided in a hospital setting where pre- and/or post-treatment infusions and/or emergency management can be more easily coordinated.

Table 3.2 Measures for management of post-operative oral bleeding.

Local/systemic	Category	Examples	Notes
Local	Absorbable collagen	Gelfoam (Pfizer), Surgicel (Ethicon)	Can be useful for alterations in both primary/secondary hemostasis
	Topical thrombin	Recothrom (Zymogenetics)	Technique sensitive, can be useful for persistent mucosal bleeding when other measures fail
	Antifibrinolytic agents	Tranexemic acid mouthwash (not commercially available in the United States) ε-aminocaproic acid syrup (Amicar)	Can be used topically (rinse or soaked gauze) or as a swish and swallow for both topical and systemic effects
Systemic	Factor replacement	Cryoprecipitate	Hemophilia A and vWD if factor or DDAVP unavailable
		Recombinant factor	Indicated for hemophilias
		Fresh frozen plasma (FFP)	Indicated for advanced liver disease, effective for hemophilia
		Desmopressin (DDAVP)	Hemophilia A, vWD; temporarily increases FVIII and vWF levels
	Vitamin K	Phytonadione	Reverses effects of warfarin, given intravenously
	Antifibrinolytic	ε-aminocaproic acid (Amicar)Tranexamic acid (Cyklokapron)	Blocks plasminogen, decreases plasmin formation, and inhibits fibrinolysis; indicated for hemophilias

3.2.3.2 *Local measures*

Local hemostatic measures should always be utilized and oftentimes provide sufficient control without any systemic intervention. The use of a higher concentration of vasoconstrictor-containing local anesthetic, such as 2% lidocaine with 1:50,000 epinephrine, can provide excellent localized hemostasis and may be sufficient for minor surgical procedures, such as a punch biopsy. Absorbable hemostatic materials made of collagen (e.g., Gelfoam) can be easily packed into extraction sockets, helping to initiate and stabilize the clot. Absorbable sponge-like materials are particularly easy to manipulate and pack into extraction sites (Figure 3.7). When there is a soft tissue wound that can be closed surgically, the use of sutures can be beneficial in reducing the size of the clot and providing greater clot stability. In some cases, surgical sites may be initially packed with a hemostatic material, then sutured, providing much greater bleeding control compared with either intervention separately. Topical thrombin converts fibrinogen to fibrin and can be applied directly to an area of bleeding, acting as an immediate glue-like substance, although this material can be difficult to work with and is fairly technique sensitive.

3.2.3.3 *Medication-induced platelet disorders*

Patients taking ASA, NSAIDs, and ADP inhibitors are at very low risk of having oral bleeding complications. When patients are taking these medications for prevention of thromboembolic disease, the increased risk of a thromboembolic event if the medication is

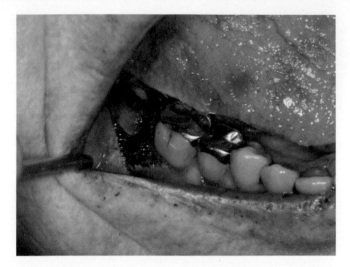

Figure 3.7 Use of Surgicel packed into a site of persistent subgingival bone bleeding following a crown-lengthening procedure in a patient with severe von Willebrand disease. Bleeding had persisted despite extensive prophylactic and post-operative systemic measures.

discontinued far outweighs any potential risk for an episode of uncontrolled bleeding that can otherwise be managed if necessary. If persistent bleeding and/or oozing are noted, local measures should be applied, although in most cases pressure with gauze is sufficient to obtain adequate hemostasis.

3.2.3.4 *Thrombocytopenia*

Patients with a platelet count greater than 50,000 cells/mm³ will generally not require additional platelets for adequate hemostasis prior to oral surgical procedures, even multiple extractions. Primary hemostasis diminishes as the platelet count drops below 50,000 cells/mm³, and below 20,000 cells/mm³ there is serious risk of bleeding. There is currently no therapeutic growth factor that consistently and reliably increases levels of circulating platelets, such as is the case with recombinant erythropoietin for patients with chronic anemia. Patients with severe thrombocytopenia are transfused with platelets as needed to maintain a count between 10,000 and 20,000 cells/mm³ to minimize risk of spontaneous hemorrhage. One unit of platelets will typically raise the platelet count by 5,000–10,000 cells/mm³. In patients requiring platelets prior to oral surgical procedures, six units are often given to ensure that the count rises to at least 50,000 cells/mm³. Platelets should be transfused as close as possible to the time of the scheduled procedure.

While post-operative oozing is not uncommon in patients taking acetasylic acid and NSAIDs, local measures are usually effective in controlling bleeding. These medications are not typically discontinued prior to surgical procedures, especially when taken for their anti-thrombotic properties.

3.2.3.5 *Hemophilia A and B*

Pre-operative factor levels should be at least 40–50% of normal to minimize risk of post-operative bleeding. The patient's hematologist should always be consulted in advance, and treatment requires careful coordination. Factor levels of at least 20–30% are required to safely deliver block injections due to the risk of developing a dissecting hematoma, which

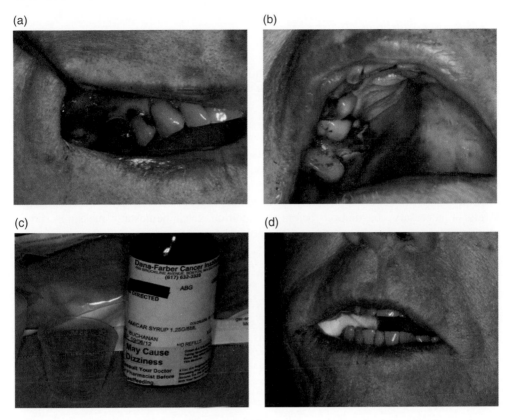

Figure 3.8 Prolonged and uncontrolled gingival bleeding in a patient with advanced leukemia despite packing of Gelfoam (b). Gauze soaked in aminocaproic acid syrup was used locally for effective control of bleeding (c and d).

can potentially lead to airway obstruction. Use of vasoconstrictors and slow delivery of the local anesthetic reduces this risk, and if a hematoma develops, use of ice packs may be sufficient, although further factor replacement may be necessary.

Depending on the severity of hemophilia, management may include any of the following: local measures alone, DDAVP, factor replacement, and/or antifibrinolytic agents. DDAVP may raise FVIII levels sufficiently in patients with mild hemophilia A to preclude the need for factor replacement. When factor replacement is necessary, it should be given as close as possible to the time of the procedure, and in situations where extensive bleeding can be anticipated, for example following multiple extractions, post-operative replacement may also be required. For patients with inhibitors to factor, local measures become even more critical, as even high levels of factor replacement may not adequately restore function.

Systemically administered antifibrinolytic agents include ε-aminocaproic acid (Amicar) and tranexamic acid. Both agents block the conversion of plasminogen to plasmin, in effect maintaining or stabilizing the clot. Use of these agents post-operatively can reduce the amount of factor replacement required. Aminocaproic acid is available as a 250/mL solution that can be swished and swallowed, or soaked in gauze and placed at the site of bleeding, for management of post-operative bleeding (Figure 3.8). Tranexamic acid is only available via IV administration. The need for antifibrinolytic therapy should be determined in consultation with a hematologist.

3.2.3.6 *von Willebrand disease*

With mild cases of vWD, which represents the vast majority of affected patients, most oral bleeding can be managed with local measures alone. In some cases DDAVP alone may be sufficient to adequately raise FVIII levels, while in more severe cases factor replacement is required. Depending on the clinical severity of vWD, management may require careful coordination with a hematologist.

3.2.3.7 *Liver disease*

The risk of post-operative bleeding in patients with advanced liver disease is dependent on the extent of organ dysfunction. Consultation with the patient's hepatologist and careful review of laboratory values are essential prior to performing invasive procedures. When indicated, infusion with FFP just prior to the dental procedure effectively restores sufficient levels of necessary coagulation factors. In addition, local hemostatic measures should always be taken, and post-operative antifibrinolytic therapy may be required.

3.3 Suggested literature

Galanis T, Thomson L, Palladino M, Merli GJ. New oral anticoagulants. J Thromb Thrombolysis 2011;31:310–320.

Gómez-Moreno G, Cutando-Soriano A, Arana C, Scully C. Hereditary blood coagulation disorders: Management and dental treatment. J Dent Res 2005;84:978–985.

Gupta A, Epstein JB, Cabay RJ. Bleeding disorders of importance in dental care and related patient management. J Can Dent Assoc 2007 Feb;73:77–83.

4 Potential for Infection

4.0 INTRODUCTION

The immune system is the primary defense mechanism against potential pathogens, including bacteria, viruses, fungi, and parasites. To prevent infection, the body possesses a complex, layered defense system that begins with physical barriers to foreign insult (e.g., skin, mucous). If a pathogen breaches these physical barriers, activation of the *innate immune system* occurs, triggering an immediate, non-specific response by leukocytes (white blood cells) including macrophages, neutrophils, and dendritic cells as well as antimicrobial proteins such as lysozyme, defensins, and the complement system. Next, activation of the *adaptive* or *acquired immune system* generates a pathogen-specific humoral (B-cell) and cell-mediated (T-cell) immune response that results in long-term memory of specific pathogens. Normal immune response is dependent on leukocytes, and alterations in the number or function of these cells may render a patient susceptible to infection.

Oral health care providers manage dental diseases and are therefore responsible for preventing and/or eliminating bacterial infections of both pulpal and periodontal etiology. Further, prior to performing invasive dental treatment, the oral health care provider must consider a patient's risk for bacterial infection to determine whether the procedure is safe and/or necessary, and whether prophylactic and/or post-operative measures are warranted. This chapter will discuss evaluation of patient risk for oral bacterial infection associated with dental treatment; however, these principles generally apply to oral viral and fungal infections as well (see chapter 7).

4.1 Medical conditions associated with an increased risk of oral infection

A number of medical conditions are characterized by quantitative and/or qualitative compromise of the immune system. In addition to the disorders discussed in this chapter, other conditions warrant consideration, such as autoimmune and immune-mediated conditions, which may be associated with an increased risk of oral infection primarily due to the secondary effects of immunosuppressive therapies (see chapter 11). Further, a number of

Risk Assessment and Oral Diagnostics in Clinical Dentistry, First Edition.
Dena J. Fischer, Nathaniel S. Treister and Andres Pinto.

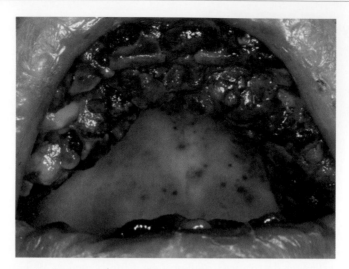

Figure 4.1 Gingival infiltrate of leukemic cells in a 42-year-old female recently diagnosed with acute lymphocytic leukemia.

other rare disorders such as cyclic neutropenia and common variable immune deficiency (CVID) are associated with an increased risk of infection.

4.1.1 Hematologic malignancies

Patients with hematologic malignancies (e.g., leukemia and lymphoma) are at a significantly increased risk of developing infections due to primary and secondary immunosuppression. Hematologic malignancies are characterized by clonal proliferation and dysfunction of a specific hematopoietic cell line. The bone marrow, lymphatic system, peripheral circulation, and major organs may be involved, and foci of malignant cells may also be present in the oral cavity (Figure 4.1). Overproduction of malignant cells may lead to deficits in normal-functioning leukocytes and in some cases cytopenias (reduction of other blood cells). Management of hematologic malignancies typically includes high-dose intensive chemotherapy with or without hematopoietic stem cell transplantation (HSCT), which also significantly increases the risk of infection (see chapter 10).

4.1.1.1 *Leukemia*
Leukemia is characterized by an abnormal proliferation of white blood cells (WBCs). This disease can affect almost any age group, although some subtypes are more prevalent later in life (e.g., chronic lymphocytic leukemia), while others affect predominantly children (e.g., acute lymphoblastic leukemia). Leukemias are further subdivided by cell lineage. *Lymphoblastic* or *lymphocytic leukemias* (acute lymphoblastic leukemia, chronic lymphocytic leukemia) affect the bone marrow cells that differentiate into lymphocytes (B-cells and T-cells), while *myelogenous leukemias* (acute myelogenous leukemia, chronic myelogenous leukemia) affect the bone marrow cells that differentiate into red blood cells, platelets, and other types of WBCs. Leukemias are characterized by an abnormally elevated white blood cell count, though these cells are highly dysfunctional and therefore patients are at significant risk for infection. In addition, thrombocytopenia (decreased platelet count) may occur, resulting in an increased risk of bleeding (see chapter 3).

Treatment for leukemia involves high-dose induction chemotherapy followed by multiple sessions of consolidation chemotherapy, although the specific regimen and sequence varies depending on the underlying diagnosis (see chapter 10). Periods of significant and in some cases prolonged myelosuppression are expected during treatment (Section 4.2.1). Depending on the specific leukemia diagnosis and response to initial chemotherapy, patients may undergo HSCT, potentially resulting in profound immunosuppression and very high risk for infection during and following transplantation.

4.1.1.2   *Lymphoma*

Lymphoma is a malignant proliferation of lymphocytes that presents as solid tumors. Lymph nodes are most commonly affected, resulting in lymphadenopathy and complications secondary to bulky disease, but lymphoma can also occur in other locations, including the oral cavity *(extranodal lymphoma)*. The World Health Organization categorizes lymphomas by cell type into the following groups: (a) Hodgkin lymphoma, (b) B-cell neoplasms, (c) T-cell and natural killer (NK) cell neoplasms, and (d) immunodeficiency-associated lymphoproliferative disorders. Hodgkin lymphoma is characterized by the proliferation of mature, dysfunctional B-cells and primarily affects adults, with peaks in the second and eighth decades of life. Non-Hodgkin lymphomas are characterized by malignant proliferation of B-lymphocytes (85% of cases) or T-lymphocytes or NK cells (15% of cases). Lymphoma or other lymphoproliferative disorders may also be associated with conditions characterized by immunosuppression, such as human immunodeficiency virus (HIV) infection or organ transplant recipients.

Chemotherapy is the mainstay of treatment, with occasional use of adjuvant radiotherapy. Patients may also be treated with hematopoietic stem cell transplantation (see chapter 10).

4.1.1.3   *Multiple myeloma*

Multiple myeloma is a malignancy of clonal plasma cells that secrete elevated amounts of immunoglobulin (antibodies) or fragments of immunoglobulin. Malignant cells proliferate in bones, where they cause lytic lesions and bone pain and increase the risk for pathologic fractures. Multiple myeloma is more common in males and African-Americans, with median survival ranging from 4 to 7 years. Increased risk of infection results from reduced hematopoiesis as well as decreased production and increased destruction of normal antibodies. Other common complications include hypercalcemia, renal failure, thrombocytopenia, and anemia. In addition to multiagent chemotherapy protocols and autologous HSCT, high-dose intravenous antiresorptive therapy is a mainstay of myeloma management. Antiresorptive agents are intended to prevent skeletal fractures but have been associated with osteonecrosis of the jaw and can lead to secondary infectious complications (see chapter 10).

4.1.2   *Aplastic anemia*

Aplastic anemia is an acquired or inherited hematologic deficiency affecting all marrow lineages. Aplastic anemia manifests clinically as pancytopenia, with decreases in WBC, red blood cell, and platelet counts (see chapter 2). Risk of infection and bleeding is increased proportionally to the cell counts. Aplastic anemia is largely idiopathic but has been associated with a number of etiologic factors including environmental exposure to chemicals or ionizing radiation, medications, autoimmune disease, and genetic syndromes (e.g., dyskeratosis congenita). Treatment for aplastic anemia includes immunosuppressive therapy, targeted immune therapy, androgen therapy, and, in severe cases, allogeneic HSCT.

Table 4.1 Oral manifestations of HIV disease.

Infectious	Viral – HSV and VZV: recurrent mucosal/skin eruption – HPV: mucosal papillomas – CMV-associated ulceration – EBV: oral hairy leukoplakia Fungal (candidiasis, deep fungal: histoplasmosis, coccidiomycosis) Bacterial (acute necrotizing gingivitis/periodontitis)
Neoplastic	Non-Hodgkin lymphoma Squamous cell carcinoma Kaposi sarcoma
Immune-mediated	Diffuse parotid enlargement Major aphthous ulcers

4.1.3 HIV infection

Human immunodeficiency virus (HIV) was estimated to affect thirty-four million people worldwide in 2010. The target for HIV is the CD4+ T-cell, with viremia gradually depleting CD4+ T-cells, weakening the immune system, and rendering patients susceptible to life-threatening opportunistic infections. Acquired immunodeficiency syndrome (AIDS) is defined by the World Health Organization as documented HIV infection in combination with a CD4+ T-cell count below 200 cells/mm^3, a CD4+ T-cell percentage less than 15%, or an AIDS-defining illness (e.g., deep fungal infection, HIV-encephalopathy, lymphoma, disseminated tuberculosis). The diagnosis of HIV is performed using a serum-based enzyme-linked immunoassay (ELISA) and confirmatory Western blot. An FDA-approved salivary-based rapid test for infection is available to all health care providers and may provide a simple alternative for screening for HIV disease. This test can be utilized in out-patient settings for high-risk individuals, and when positive, confirmatory serum testing is recommended due to its higher specificity.

Management of HIV infection is based on a combination of nucleoside and non-nucleo-side reverse transcriptase inhibitors, protease inhibitors, cellular entry blockers, and inte-grase inhibitors. With the inception of highly active antiretroviral therapy (HAART) in the mid-1990s, HIV disease for those with access to therapy has become a chronic and largely manageable disease. HIV disease monitoring is based on periodic (at least once every 6 months) testing for CD4+ T-cell count, CD8+ T-cell count, and HIV viral load. Decreased CD4+ T-cell and abnormal CD4+/CD8+ counts are markers for disease progression, and a decreased CD4+ T-cell count below 500 cells/mm^3 indicates significant immune dysfunction and increased risk for infection. Measurements of viral load may also be utilized to assess disease progression or response to treatment. Viral load is determined by measuring plasma levels of HIV RNA, with detectable copy numbers indicating response or progression based on an individual's previous numbers and overall trends.

There are numerous infectious and non-infectious oral manifestations of HIV disease, and the presence of these conditions may signify disease progression or inadequate response to therapy (Table 4.1). Acute necrotizing periodontitis occurs with increased frequency in patients with HIV disease and is characterized by generalized gingival ulceration and necrosis, pain, and halitosis (Figure 4.2). Oral candidiasis is the most common opportunistic infection in HIV-positive patients (see chapter 7). Deep fungal infections, such as *Aspergillus* or *Coccidioides immitis*, develop infrequently in the oral cavity, typically presenting as a

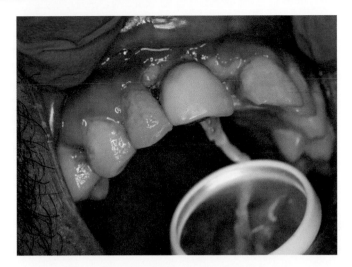

Figure 4.2 Acute necrotizing ulcerative periodontitis in a 37-year-old AIDS patient with a CD4+ T-cell count of 2 cells/mm³.

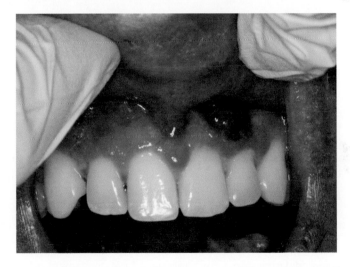

Figure 4.3 Prominent nodular maxillary oral involvement in a 26-year-old male with advanced AIDS and multifocal disseminated Kaposi sarcoma.

solitary ulceration in severely immunocompromised patients. Herpes virus infections are relatively common in HIV-positive patients. Recrudescent orofacial herpes simplex virus (HSV) infection presents as herpes labialis or as intraoral ulcerative lesions (see chapter 7). Reactivation of varicella zoster virus (VZV) and cytomegalovirus (CMV) intraorally or extraorally occurs much less frequently and may correlate with disease progression. Oral hairy leukoplakia is an Epstein-Barr virus (EBV)–associated condition characterized by bilateral asymptomatic white plaques on the ventrolateral surfaces of the tongue (see chapter 7). Kaposi sarcoma is a neoplasm associated with human herpes virus 8 and frequently presents as intraoral pigmented plaques and nodular lesions (Figure 4.3). Squamous papillomas are caused by human papilloma virus (HPV) infection and may

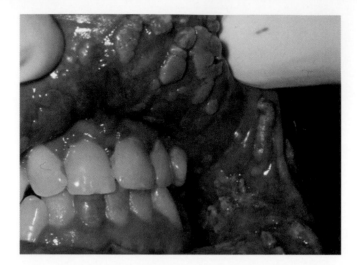

Figure 4.4   Multiple nodular papillomas in a 46-year-old HIV-positive male who was noncompliant with antiretroviral therapy.

present in multiple areas throughout the oral cavity (Figure 4.4). Recurrent major aphthous ulcers can be quite severe and are highly associated with a suppressed CD4+ T-cell count.

4.1.4   Endocrine disorders

Alterations in the endocrine system can lead to suppression of the immune system and an increased susceptibility to infection (see chapter 5). Diabetes mellitus is an endocrinopathy characterized by impaired glucose metabolism and hyperglycemia, which when uncontrolled leads to impaired neutrophil motility and function and an increased risk for infection. In addition, both primary (e.g., Cushing syndrome) and secondary (i.e., due to prolonged corticosteroid therapy) adrenal disorders can adversely impact the function and quantity of immune cells, predisposing the individual to infection.

4.2   Medications associated with an increased risk of infection

The most common cause of leukopenia (decreased WBC count) is iatrogenic, resulting from the use of immunomodulating or cytotoxic therapies for management of immune-mediated diseases, transplantation, or cancer. This mechanism of bone marrow suppression is typically dose-related and may vary with continued administration of the drug. Idiosyncratic reactions to a number of non-immunosuppressive medications, such as carbamazepine, may also result in leukopenia and in severe cases bone marrow failure (Table 4.2).

4.2.1   Chemotherapy

Cancer chemotherapy is associated with a significantly increased risk of infection due to unintended but expected bone marrow toxicity. The effect of chemotherapy on WBCs is dependent on the particular agent, dose, intensity, and frequency of administration. Cytoreductive chemotherapy, which is intended to reduce the population of tumor cells, also causes a decrease in the WBC count, usually within 2 weeks of initiation of treatment. Treatment "cycles" are typically 3–4 weeks in duration, and WBC counts recover to normal levels in between cycles (see chapter 10). With some cancer chemotherapy protocols, the infection risk is so great that

Table 4.2 Select medications associated with leukopenia.

Class	Examples	Mechanism
Antibiotics	Minocycline, Amoxicillin	Hypersensitivity response
Anticonvulsants	Lamotrigine, Divalproex sodium, Carbamazepine	Bone marrow suppression
Antidepressants	Bupropion hydrochloride	Unknown
Antiemetic	Promethazine hydrochloride, Chlorpromazine	Bone marrow suppression
Antifungals	Terbinafine, Fluconazole	Bone marrow suppression
Antigout	Colchicine	Direct toxicity of WBC
Anti-inflammatory	Sulfasalazine	Bone marrow suppression
Antimalarial	Pyrimethamine	Bone marrow suppression
Antipsychotics	Clozapine	Autoimmune or direct toxicity
Immunomodulating agents	Cyclosporine, Tacrolimus, Azathioprine, Mycophenolate mofetil, Sirolimus, Corticosteroids, Methotrexate	Bone marrow suppression
Muscle relaxants	Methocarbamol, Carisoprodol	Unknown

patients are placed on prophylactic antimicrobial therapy, and the schedule and dose of chemotherapy may be modified if there is unexpectedly profound bone marrow suppression.

4.2.2   Corticosteroid therapy and other immunomodulatory agents

Corticosteroids and other immunomodulatory drugs are used to treat a wide range of diseases (Table 4.2). Patients with autoimmune or immune-mediated diseases and organ transplant recipients often require long-term immunomodulatory therapy. These medications have both quantitative (decrease WBC counts) and qualitative (inhibit leukocyte function) activities. With corticosteroid therapy, both the total daily dose and the overall duration of therapy are important factors to consider when performing risk assessment. Patients on long-term high-dose corticosteroid therapy (i.e., 0.5–1 mg/kg/day of prednisone/ prednisolone) who are planned to undergo invasive dental procedures may be at risk for developing oral infection. Immunomodulatory therapy is usually administered in low or moderate doses and for extended periods of time. The impact of immunomodulatory therapy on oral infection risk is uncertain, and although there may be a long-term decrease in the WBC count, there appears to be minimal effect on the functional aspects of these cells.

4.3   Tests for evaluating infection risk

4.3.1   Basic tests of white blood cells

The WBC count is included as part of a complete blood count (see chapter 2). Normal values range from 4,000 to 11,000 cells/mm^3 (see Alert Box 2.3). Leukocytosis may occur during acute infection and hemorrhage, or as a physiologic response to stress, exercise, or temperature changes. Infection stimulates the production of WBCs as part of the immune response, resulting in a temporary leukocytosis. Leukopenia may develop secondary to infection, hematologic disorders (e.g., bone marrow failure disorders and malignancies), immune-mediated diseases, and medications.

Table 4.3 WBC differential values.

Cell type	Normal ranges	% of WBC	Clinical significance of values
Neutrophils	3,000–7,000 cells/mm^3	54–62%	Increased: – prevalence of immature cells (bands), referred to as a "left shift" – prevalence of mature and multinucleated cells, referred to as a "right shift" – rule out infection Decreased: duration of neutropenia is the most important risk factor for infection *Panic value* < 500 cells/mm^3
Eosinophils	50–500 cells/mm^3	1–3%	Increased: associated with parasitic infection, endocrine disease, allergy, and malignancy Decreased: associated with infections, systemic shock *Panic value* < 50 cells/mm^3
Basophils	20–50 cells/mm^3	0–0.75%	Increased: associated with chronic myeloid leukemia Decreased: associated with Cushing syndrome, rheumatic fever
Monocytes	100–500 cells/mm^3	3–7%	Increased: associated with infection, hematologic malignancy, endocarditis Decreased: associated with autoimmune disorders, tuberculosis, malaria
Lymphocytes	1,500–4,000 cells/mm^3	25–33%	Increased: associated with acute viral infection, hematologic malignancy Decreased: associated with medications, immunosupression, renal disease *Panic value* < 100 cells/mm^3

4.3.1.1 *WBC differential count*

The WBC differential count is reported as an absolute count or as a proportion of each type of leukocyte within the total WBC count (Table 4.3). Neutrophils are the most numerous type of leukocyte and constitute a primary defense against bacterial invasion. Perhaps the most important WBC differential test for assessing bacterial infection risk is the absolute neutrophil count (ANC), which measures the total number of neutrophils and includes mature neutrophils (segmented neutrophils, account for 50–60% of total WBC) and bands (immature neutrophils, account for 3–5% of total WBC). An ANC that is below 1,000 neutrophils/mm^3 predisposes patients to the development of infection, and this risk increases dramatically when the ANC is 500 cells/mm^3 or below (Alert Box 4.1; Figure 4.5). The

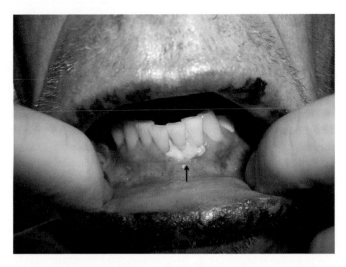

Figure 4.5 Gingival neutropenic ulceration in a young male being treated for acute myelogenous leukemia with profound neutropenia. Note the lack of marginal erythema, and note labial ulcerations and crusting consistent with recrudescent herpes simplex infection.

overall duration of neutropenia is also an important consideration, as a patient with a very low ANC (i.e., below 100 cells/mm^3) for 1–2 days with quick count recovery is at a much lower risk for infection compared to a patient with a higher but still critically low ANC that persists for several weeks.

Eosinophils contain histamine-laden granules and contribute to acute allergic responses. Eosinophilia most commonly indicates an allergic response or parasitic disease, though elevated eosinophils may occur in the presence of rheumatic disease, Addison disease, chronic myeloid leukemia, or myeloproliferative disorders. Eosinopenia may also develop secondary to an increase in adrenal steroid production secondary to chronic stress, Cushing syndrome, or ACTH therapy (see chapter 5).

Basophils are a small component of the total leukocyte count. Basophilia may indicate a parasitic infection, allergic disorder, leukemia, or myeloproliferative disorder. Basopenia can be seen in the context of chemotherapy, radiation, prolonged corticosteroid therapy, rheumatic fever, or hyperthyroidism.

Monocytes are involved in phagocytosis and antigen presentation. Monocytosis may occur with acute bacterial infections, leukemia, or lymphoma. A decreased monocyte count has been linked to stress, acute infections, and prolonged corticosteroid therapy.

The lymphocyte differential count incorporates T- and B-lymphocytes and NK cells. Quantification of lymphocyte subpopulations is not performed as part of a routine CBC. Lymphocytosis is common in viral infections and occurs with some bacterial infections and hematologic malignancies. Lymphopenia may develop in the context of immune deficiency/immunomodulating disorders or may be caused iatrogenically by immunosuppressive medications. Patients with severe lymphopenia are highly susceptible to viral and fungal infection.

4.3.2   Adjunctive tests

Additional testing may be helpful to assess immune function in some individuals. While these tests are generally ordered by specialist physicians, oral health care providers should be familiar with their use and the interpretation of their results. Bone marrow sampling includes biopsy and aspiration and can be utilized to evaluate hematopoiesis and detect malignant cells in the marrow. This test is performed routinely in patients undergoing treatment for hematologic disease to assess response to therapy.

Flow cytometry is a test used to determine the composition of circulating lymphocyte populations, and while it does not directly assess risk for infection, test findings may be considered in determining overall immune status and function. Flow cytometry uses peripheral blood and is based on fluorescence-labeled antibodies specific to lymphocyte surface markers. Conditions for which flow cytometry may be useful in establishing a diagnosis include hereditary spherocytosis, idiopathic thrombocytopenia, and hematologic malignancies.

Neutrophil function testing assesses chemotactic and/or bactericidal activity. Testing for qualitative defects is generally ordered by a hematologist or immunologist and involves microscopic examination of granular cell morphology, flow cytometry, and genetic testing for known mutations that interfere with normal function. The American Society of Hematology recommends neutrophil function testing be ordered in patients with a history of two or more systemic infections, successive respiratory infections (sinusitis or pneumonia), onset of infections in unusual organs (e.g., liver, brain), and generalized infections with rare pathogens such as *Nocardia* and *Aspergillus*.

4.4   Implications of abnormal wbc tests on provision of oral care

Invasive dental procedures include any intervention that involves manipulation of the periodontium (e.g., scaling and root planing, surgeries), pulp chamber (e.g., endodontic therapy with or without instrumentation beyond the apex), alveolar bone (e.g., extractions, crown lengthening, implant placement), or mucosa (e.g., soft tissue biopsy). All of these procedures are associated with tissue trauma and hemorrhage and may cause an increased risk of oral infection. The risk is greater for more invasive procedures; for example, a surgical extraction that requires removal of bone is a higher-risk procedure than a simple extraction of a periodontally-involved mobile tooth.

For most restorative dental treatments, simple periodontal procedures and atraumatic extractions, the risk of infection is very low and hematologic testing is not usually indicated. In general, physician consultation is recommended prior to performing invasive dental procedures on all patients who are at increased risk for oral infection. Further, in patients with known hematologic disease or recent history (within 1 year) of HSCT, consultation with the patient's hematologist/oncologist is warranted prior to performing any dental procedures.

In patients who are known to be at increased risk for oral infection, WBC testing with differential count should be ordered prior to performing invasive procedures. The risk for post-operative bacterial infections generally correlates with the neutrophil count. Therefore the ANC is a highly useful lab value that can be used to assess infection risk and help determine whether or not antibiotic prophylaxis and/or post-operative coverage are warranted (Alert Box 4.1). When urgent care is required in the presence of significant neutropenia (ANC less than 1,000 cells/mm^3) or primary hematologic disease with quantitative or qualitative neutropenia (ANC less than 2,000 cells/mm^3), pre-operative antibiotics should be started 1–2 days prior to the procedure (if not already prescribed for infection management), followed by at least a 7- to 10-day post-operative course with frequent monitoring (see Table 7.2). Whenever possible, dental treatment should be deferred in patients with severe neutropenia. When patients on cycled chemotherapy require an invasive dental procedure—for example, if a patient develops irreversible pulpitis during cancer treatment—the dental procedure should be scheduled to correspond

Alert Box 4.1   Absolute neutrophil count and infection risk.

Risk level	ANC count (cells/mm³)	Medical consultation recommended?	Interventions
Low (normal)	3,000–7,000	No	None
Moderate	< 2,000	Yes	Consult physician concerning risk of infection if patient has known hematologic disease
High	< 1,000	Yes	Consider perioperative (pre-operative dose and 1 week post-operative dose) antibiotic coverage in patients who are immunosuppressed or have autoimmune disease
Panic	< 500	Yes	Perioperative antibiotic coverage is indicated

with WBC count recovery if possible. This scenario allows for 2 weeks of healing following the procedure before the counts are once again depressed in the next chemotherapy cycle.

4.5   Antibiotic prophylaxis for dental procedures

Bacteremia is defined as the presence of bacteria in the bloodstream, which occurs transiently on a daily basis and is rarely associated with any medical complications in healthy individuals. Bacteremia arising from oral sources occurs following tooth brushing, flossing, and mastication, and this transient bacteremia is resolved by an intact immune response, which prevents bacterial seeding at distant sites (e.g., the heart). In the presence of endothelial injury or damaged or prosthetic cardiac valves, there is an increased risk of hematologic seeding and development of valvular vegetations.

The most frequently isolated microorganisms during episodes of bacteremia include the *streptococci* family (*Viridans* sp.), *staphylococci*, and the *HACEK* group (*Haemophilus, Actinobacillus, Cardiobacterium, Eikenella*, and *Klebsiella*). Because many of these organisms are known to be components of the oral microflora, dental procedures have been linked to the onset of cardiac and non-cardiac complications of systemic bacteremia, including bacterial seeding of cardiac valves and prosthetic joints. Prophylactic administration of antibiotics prior to dental procedures in patients thought to be at increased risk has been a common practice in medicine and dentistry.

4.5.1   Cardiac complications

Bacterial endocarditis, or "infective endocarditis," is a serious medical complication that can arise secondary to bacteremia. Endocarditis is a life-threatening condition defined as inflammation of the heart that may affect both the valves and surrounding tissues (pericardium) and results in significant morbidity and mortality. The incidence of endocarditis is between 2.6 and 7 cases per 100,000, and up to 30% involve prosthetic cardiac valves. Management includes intensive long-term antibiotic therapy, and in some cases surgery to repair or replace damaged valves. Patients at risk include those with endothelial damage, prosthetic or repaired valves, a history of intravenous drug use (due to exposure to dermatologic pathogens such as *Staphylococcus aureus*), and previous episodes of endocarditis.

Bacteria from oral sources are commonly believed to be responsible for a significant number of cases of bacterial endocarditis, based on the identification of bacteria normally found in the oral microflora isolated from blood cultures. Bacteremia composed of oral flora has been assumed to result from dental treatment, and this has been the justification for prescribing prophylactic antibiotics prior to dental visits. However, it remains unclear what role, if any, bacteremia specifically from oral sources plays in the development of endocarditis. Furthermore, it is now well recognized that daily bacteremias occur on a far more frequent basis than dental visit–associated bacteremias, suggesting that a patient's overall oral hygiene status is probably the most important factor to be addressed in high-risk individuals.

4.5.2 Prosthetic joint complications

Joint replacements are performed to restore function in patients with osteoarthritic or rheumatoid disorders. More than 400,000 joint replacements are performed in the United States every year, with the majority being hips and knees. Late joint infection (3–24 months post-surgery) due to hematologic bacterial seeding of artificial joints is uncommon, affecting approximately 2% of hip replacements and 1% of knee replacements. However, costs and morbidity associated with treatment of this complication are extremely high, and there is a high risk of septicemia from late bacterial joint infections. Patients who have poor healing (see chapter 5), autoimmune disease, or those on long-term immunosuppressive therapies are at a higher risk for developing prosthetic joint complications. Similar to endocarditis, bacteria from oral sources are believed to play a role in the development of late prosthetic joint infections, in part based on the identification of oral bacteria in infected joints. Nevertheless, there is no rigorous systematic analysis of the published evidence on the cumulative incidence of joint infections caused by bacteria of oral origin and the causal relationship with the development of late prosthetic joint infections.

4.5.3 Recommendations for antibiotic prophylaxis

The American Heart Association (AHA) has developed (and continuously updates) guidelines for the use of antibiotic prophylaxis prior to invasive dental procedures for the prevention of endocarditis. The most recent AHA recommendations, published in 2007, describe any procedure that involves manipulation of gingival tissues, perforation of the oral mucosa, or manipulation of the periapical region of teeth as a risk factor for significant bacteremia. Antibiotic prophylaxis is currently recommended for patients with a prosthetic cardiac valve or prosthetic material used for valve repair, congenital unrepaired cyanotic heart disease, cyanotic heart disease with prosthetic material repaired within the last 6 months, and those who have undergone cardiac transplantation with residual valvular dysfunction (Table 4.4). The oral health provider should follow published AHA guidelines and establish the need for antibiotic prophylaxis in consultation with the patient's physician (Table 4.5).

The American Association of Orthopedic Surgeons (AAOS) and the ADA jointly published guidelines in 2003 for antibiotic prophylaxis in patients with prosthetic joints. These guidelines recommend the use of prophylactic antibiotics (following the recommendations for drug choice and dosing put forth in the AHA guidelines) prior to invasive dental procedures in patients who have received an artificial joint replacement within the previous

Table 4.4   Indications for antibiotic prophylaxis prior to invasive dental procedures for the prevention of infective endocarditis.*,†

Previous history of infectious endocarditis
Cardiac transplant with newly developed valvulopathy
Unrepaired congenital heart disease
Repaired congenital heart disease within the first 6 months
Repaired congenital heart disease with defects at site of repair
Prosthetic cardiac valve replacement or repair

*Antibiotic prophylaxis is suggested for all dental procedures that involve manipulation of the gingival tissues or periapical tissues that include violation of mucosal integrity.
†Adapted from: Wilson W, Taubert KA, Gewitz M, et al. Prevention of infective endocarditis: Guidelines from the American Heart Association: A guideline from the American Heart Association Rheumatic Fever, Endocarditis, and Kawasaki Disease Committee, Council on Cardiovascular Disease in the Young, and the Council on Clinical Cardiology, Council on Cardiovascular Surgery and Anesthesia, and the Quality of Care and Outcomes Research Interdisciplinary Working Group. Circulation 2007;116:1736–1754.

Table 4.5   Recommended antibiotics for the prevention of infective endocarditis in adults.*

Route	Antibiotic	One dose (within 1 hour prior to dental procedure)
Oral	Amoxicillin	2 g
If not able to take oral medication	Ampicillin or Cefazolin	2 g IV or IM
	Ceftriaxone	1 g IV or IM
Allergic to penicillin or ampicillin	Cephalexin	2 g
	Clindamycin	600 mg
	Clarithromycin or Azithromycin	500 mg
Allergic to penicillin or ampicillin (not able to take oral medication)	Cefazolin or Ceftriaxone	1 g IV or IM
	Clindamycin	600 mg IV or IM

IV: Intravenous.
IM: Intramuscular.
*Adapted from: Wilson W, Taubert KA, Gewitz M, et al. Prevention of infective endocarditis: Guidelines from the American Heart Association: A guideline from the American Heart Association Rheumatic Fever, Endocarditis, and Kawasaki Disease Committee, Council on Cardiovascular Disease in the Young, and the Council on Clinical Cardiology, Council on Cardiovascular Surgery and Anesthesia, and the Quality of Care and Outcomes Research Interdisciplinary Working Group. Circulation 2007;116:1736–1754.

2 years, and in any immunosuppressed individual who has received a prosthetic joint at any time in the past. A 2010 position paper from the AAOS recommended that all patients who have received a prosthetic joint should use antibiotic prophylaxis prior to dental procedures indefinitely. A revised combined statement from the AAOS and the ADA is forthcoming. Oral health care providers should discuss specific cases with the treating orthopedic surgeon/orthopedist and refer to updated guidelines when available.

4.6   Suggested literature

American Academy of Orthopaedic Surgeons. Information statement: Antibiotic prophylaxis for bacteremia in patients with joint replacements. www.aaos.org/about/papers/advistmt/1033.asp, accessed February 1, 2012.
Antibiotic prophylaxis for dental patients with total joint replacements. American Dental Association; American Academy of Orthopedic Surgeons. JADA 2003;134:895–899.
Dale DC, Welte K. Cyclic and chronic neutropenia. Cancer Treat Res 2011;157:97–108.

Elad S, Zadik Y, Hewson I, Hovan A, Correa ME, Logan R, et al. A systematic review of viral infections associated with oral involvement in cancer patients: A spotlight on Herpesviridea. Support Care Cancer 2010;18:993–1006.

Hupp WS, Firriolo FJ, De Rossi SS. Laboratory evaluation of chronic medical conditions for dental treatment: Part III. Hematology. Compend Contin Educ Dent 2011;32:10–12, 14–18.

Narayan KM, Ali MK, del Rio C, Koplan JP, Curran J. Global noncommunicable diseases—lessons from the HIV-AIDS experience. N Engl J Med 2011;365:876–878.

Patton LL, Ranganathan K, Naidoo S, Bhayat A, Balasundaram S, Adeyemi O, Taiwo O, Speicher DJ, Chandra L. Oral lesions, HIV phenotypes, and management of HIV-related disease: Workshop 4A. Adv Dent Res 2011;23:112–116.

Williams D, Lewis M. Pathogenesis and treatment of oral candidosis. J Oral Microbiol 2011 Jan 28;3. doi: 10.3402/jom.v3i0.5771.

Wilson W, Taubert KA, Gewitz M, Lockhart PB, Baddour LM, Levison M, et al. Prevention of infective endocarditis: Guidelines from the American Heart Association: A guideline from the American Heart Association Rheumatic Fever, Endocarditis, and Kawasaki Disease Committee, Council on Cardiovascular Disease in the Young, and the Council on Clinical Cardiology, Council on Cardiovascular Surgery and Anesthesia, and the Quality of Care and Outcomes Research Interdisciplinary Working Group. Circulation 2007;116:1736–1754.

5 Potential for Poor Wound Healing

5.0 INTRODUCTION

Hard and soft tissue injury, whether due to surgical oral procedures, disease, or trauma, can cause the formation of wounds, which, if not secondarily infected, heal normally in an uncomplicated manner in healthy individuals. Surgical oral procedures typically fully heal, often without evidence of tissue injury. Inflammatory oral conditions, such as minor recurrent aphthous stomatitis and ulcerative oral lichen planus, present with recurrent painful mucosal ulcerations that may require medical intervention to promote healing but rarely result in scar formation. Orofacial trauma can range from a minor injury such as cheek biting or a pizza burn, which typically heals without complications, to more extensive injuries including facial fractures, in which healing may require surgical intervention and may be complicated by infection secondary to the introduction of foreign material into the wound.

Wound healing is a complex and highly organized process that involves coagulation (see chapter 3), acute inflammation, cellular regeneration and proliferation, and tissue remodeling. Acute inflammation is the early reaction to injury in which a vascular and cellular response removes debris and foreign bodies from the wound. Macrophages are released from the microcirculation and clear extracellular debris, fibrin, and other foreign material at the site of wound repair. Regeneration of injured tissue begins with cell replication and angiogenesis, controlled by a complex interplay of cytokines, growth factors, and other biostimulatory mediators. If wound repair is not achieved by regeneration alone, a granulation response occurs in which there is a proliferation of fibroblasts, followed by collagen deposition and organization of fibrous connective tissue, leading to scar formation. During the remodeling phase, the wound undergoes contraction and maturation, and in most cases results in clinically normal-appearing tissue.

Healing can occur through three basic mechanisms. Primary intention is the process of wound repair achieved when the wound borders are approximated (i.e., primary closure) using sutures or other techniques to keep the borders closed during healing. Secondary intention is characterized by a wound where the borders are not precisely closed, and granulation tissue replaces the gap between the two planes (i.e., secondary closure). This type of healing is generally slower than primary intention and has a greater risk of scar formation. Most dental procedures, such as extractions and gingivectomy, heal by secondary

Risk Assessment and Oral Diagnostics in Clinical Dentistry, First Edition.
Dena J. Fischer, Nathaniel S. Treister and Andres Pinto.
© 2013 John Wiley & Sons, Inc. Published 2013 by John Wiley & Sons, Inc.

Table 5.1 Risk assessment for poor wound healing.

Risk factor	Clinical information	Preventive measure	Rationale
Poorly controlled diabetes mellitus	HbA1c $\geq$ 9%; > 12% at significantly increased risk History of infections Complications of DM	Antibiotic coverage on the day of and for 7–10 days following invasive dental procedure	Poor diabetic control interferes with normal wound healing
Neutropenia	ANC < 500 cells/mm^3	Antibiotic coverage on the day of and for 7–10 days following invasive dental procedure (consider continuing until evidence of good healing)	Infection risk very high; procedures generally deferred unless urgent
Long-term corticosteroid therapy	Corticosteroid dose > 25 mg cortisol equivalent/day Discontinuation of high-dose (> 25 mg cortisol equivalent/ day) corticosteroid therapy within the past 2 weeks	Consider steroid supplementation	Prevent potential adrenal crisis that can result from surgical stress secondary to adrenal insufficiency
	High-dose ($\geq$ 0.5–1.0 mg/ kg/day prednisone/ prednisolone) long-term corticosteroid therapy	Antibiotic coverage on the day of and for 1 week following invasive dental procedure	Long-term corticosteroid therapy interferes with normal wound healing

ANC = Absolute neutrophil count.

intention. Healing through tertiary intention is the process by which the wound is initially cleaned, debrided, and observed, followed by delayed primary closure, typically 4–5 days later. Use of reconstructive tissue grafts may undergo healing with tertiary intention.

Systemic and local factors can influence wound healing. Systemic factors that can impede healing include inadequate circulation, compromised immune function, prolonged corticosteroid therapy, antiresorptive therapy, and nutritional deficiencies. Local factors that can adversely affect healing include the size and location of the wound, mechanical insult, foreign bodies such as debris and sutures, and infection, which is the single most important cause of delay in wound healing. Given the close association between healing and infection, there is some degree of unavoidable overlap with chapter 4, and therefore these two chapters should be considered in tandem. This chapter reviews the most common disorders that increase a patient's susceptibility for poor wound healing and describes diagnostic tests that can be utilized to assess risk as well as strategies for risk reduction (Table 5.1).

5.1 Diabetes mellitus

Diabetes mellitus (DM) is an endocrine disorder characterized by progressive intolerance to glucose and its impaired metabolism. Dysfunction of the pancreatic beta cells causes defects in insulin secretion (Type 1 DM), insulin action (Type 2 DM), or both, which results in sustained hyperglycemia. Impaired glucose tolerance is a pre-diabetic state of compromised blood glucose metabolism that is associated with insulin resistance and often precedes Type 2 DM. Long-term hyperglycemia leads to the development of *glycation* in which glucose binds to proteins and other molecules through a non-enzymatic process. Glycation results in neutrophil dysfunction, diminished vascular perfusion and progressive peripheral nerve damage, all of which have systemic implications and contribute to poor wound healing.

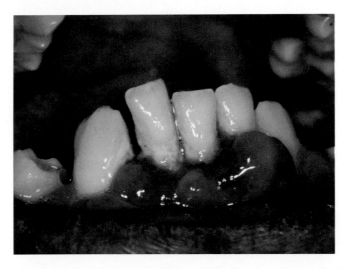

Figure 5.1   Advanced periodontal disease in a 48-year-old male with poorly controlled diabetes mellitus who presented for evaluation of multiple loose teeth and halitosis.

Long-term complications of DM include end-stage renal disease requiring hemodialysis and/or renal transplantation, coronary artery disease that increases the risk of cerebrovascular accident and myocardial infarction, retinopathy that can lead to blindness, peripheral neuropathy of the hands and feet, and chronic wounds that in some cases require amputation. Oral complications of diabetes include delayed healing and frequent oral infections. Periodontal disease can be particularly aggressive, especially in poorly-controlled diabetic patients (Figure 5.1). Diabetes is a major public health concern in the United States due to its high prevalence and long-term health consequences.

Poorly regulated insulin activity, whether due to underlying disease or inadequate management, may result in acute hypo- or hyperglycemic states. Severe hypoglycemia is characterized by diaphoresis, disorientation, dizziness, and hypotension, and requires urgent medical management (i.e., oral supplementation with simple sugars or subcutaneous administration of glucagon). Hypoglycemia episodes are not associated with impaired healing or an increased risk of infection. Acute hyperglycemia is often benign and asymptomatic; however, in cases of severe hyperglycemia (e.g., blood glucose greater than 350 mg/dL), pharmacologic supplementation is crucial and emergency medical care may be required since serious complications such as osmotic diuresis can rapidly develop.

Oral health care providers are in a unique position of being able to engage in diabetes management activities to improve health behaviors of their diabetic patients. Regular dental visits provide opportunities for education about metabolic control, diet, and medication compliance, as well as physician referral when warranted.

5.1.1   *Tests for diagnosis and monitoring of DM*

Diagnosis and monitoring of DM are assessed through plasma glucose levels. Fasting plasma glucose and the oral glucose tolerance test are used for diagnosis, random plasma glucose is used for screening and monitoring, and glycated hemoglobin (HbA1c) measures long-term diabetic control.

Table 5.2 Tests for diagnosis and monitoring of diabetes mellitus.

Indication	Test	Results		
		Normal	**Impaired glucose tolerance**	**Diabetes mellitus**
Diagnosis	Fasting plasma glucose	< 100 mg/dl	≥ 100 mg/dl and < 126 mg/dl	≥ 126 mg/dl
	Oral glucose tolerance	< 140 mg/dl	≥ 140 mg/dl	≥ 200 mg/dl
Self-management	Random plasma glucose	< 200 mg/dl	n/a	> 200 mg/dl, recheck at a later time
Long-term diabetic control	Glycated hemoglobin	*Good control* < 6.5%	*Fair control* 6.5–9%	*Poor control* > 9%

Alert Box 5.1 Casual plasma glucose values in patients with diabetes mellitus.

Risk level	Plasma glucose (mg/dL)	Medical consultation recommended?	Interventions
Low	80–110	No	None
Moderate	70–79 (low)	No	Self-monitoring of plasma glucose levels
	> 110–180 (high)	No	Self-monitoring of plasma glucose levels
High	> 200	Yes	High: Pharmacologic intervention required
	< 70	Yes	Low: Glucose supplementation required
Panic	> 400	Yes	Panic high: Emergency medical intervention required
	< 50	Yes	Panic low: Emergency glucagon supplementation required

5.1.1.1 *Diagnosis of DM: Fasting plasma glucose and oral glucose tolerance tests*

Fasting plasma glucose is a routine test performed to assess the glucose level after a period of overnight fasting. This test is used to screen patients who may have signs or symptoms related to diabetes and is performed in a medical laboratory setting after 8–12 hours of no oral intake, with the exception of daily medications and water. Two fasting glucose measurements of at least 126 mg/dL are considered diagnostic for DM (Table 5.2).

The glucose tolerance test, also referred to as the oral glucose tolerance test, is a secondary diagnostic test that is performed when a patient has an equivocal fasting glucose test (i.e., near 126 mg/dL) or borderline glycated hemoglobin (i.e., near 6.5%; section 5.1.1.3). The test evaluates the body's ability to closely regulate glucose levels. Subsequent to overnight fasting, the patient is given an oral dose of glucose (75 mg), usually in a liquid form, and plasma glucose levels are assessed at baseline, 1 hour and 2 hours following glucose intake (Table 5.2).

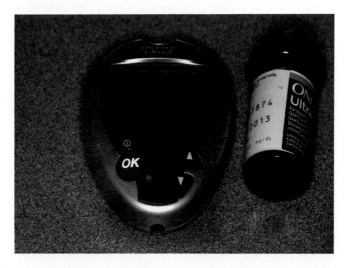

Figure 5.2   Home glucose meter for daily self-monitoring of random plasma glucose levels.

5.1.1.2   *Glucose self-monitoring: Random plasma glucose*

Random plasma glucose is defined as the measurement of circulating glucose levels at any given time throughout the day, with a normal value of 80–100 mg/dL (Table 5.2, Alert Box 5.1). The random plasma glucose can vary greatly in diabetics and depends on the time of day the measurement is taken, time elapsed since the last meal, and the schedule and dose of insulin or other diabetes-related medications. This is a common test used in diabetic patients or those with impaired glucose tolerance to monitor for hyper- /hypo-glycemic episodes, dietary compliance, and response to pharmacologic treatment. Random plasma glucose may also be utilized to screen for glucose intolerance or DM in patients who present with risk factors for diabetes.

Glucose meters for at-home random plasma glucose monitoring are available in any pharmacy (Figure 5.2). Generally, the method involves puncturing the finger to produce blood, applying blood to a test strip, placing the test strip in the meter, and analyzing. Acquiring an adequate amount of blood (at least one drop from the puncture site) and carefully following the manufacturer's instructions will minimize errors. Daily self-monitoring of plasma glucose is essential in maintaining glycemic control, improving health behaviors, and preventing long-term complications of DM.

5.1.1.3   *Diabetes control: Glycated hemoglobin (HbA1c)*

Through the process of glycation, plasma glucose binds to the amino and lysine portions of hemoglobin in red blood cells, creating HbA1c. This reaction is permanent, and the percentage of HbA1c is proportional to plasma glucose levels. Since the red blood cell lifespan is approximately 120 days, measurement of HbA1c percentage levels reflects the average plasma glucose levels during the previous 3–4 months. In healthy adults, approximately 5% of hemoglobin is glycated due to normal serum glucose levels, while periods of sustained hyperglycemia will cause increases in HbA1c levels, with 6.5% or higher constituting a diagnosis of DM (Table 5.2). Consequently, HbA1c is the most accurate measure of long-term diabetic control and response to pharmacologic intervention. When close monitoring is necessary, this test is performed at 3-month intervals. Over-the-counter devices to measure HbA1c have been recently introduced on the market.

Alert Box 5.2 Glycated hemoglobin values in patients with diabetes mellitus.

Risk Level	HbA1c values	Medical consultation recommended?	Intervention
Low	5–6.5%	No	None; minimal potential for infection, delayed healing
Moderate	7–9% (moderate control)	No	Potential for infection, delayed healing; take into consideration local and systemic factors that may contribute to infection, delayed wound healing
			Consider antibiotic coverage on the day of and for 7–10 days following invasive dental procedure
High	> 9% (poor control)	Yes	High risk for infection, delayed healing, even in the absence of additional factors that may contribute to infection, delayed wound healing
			Antibiotic coverage on the day of and for at least 7–10 days following invasive dental procedure; medical consultation to obtain better glucose control

5.1.2 Implications of abnormal tests on dental care

No specific evidence-based guidelines exist regarding provision of invasive dental treatment for patients with DM based exclusively on laboratory values. The oral health care provider should consider the laboratory testing trends in the individual diabetic patient, as well as the overall history of systemic infections, reported healing complications and the extent of planned treatment (surgical vs. non-surgical, osseous vs. mucosal) in order to perform an appropriate risk assessment. HbA1c levels that trend for several months toward poor control may justify the use of antibiotics prior to an invasive dental procedure, such as surgical treatment or deep scaling (Alert Box 5.2). Antibiotics can be started the day of the dental procedure and should be continued for at least 7–10 days. Further, the oral health care practitioner may consider delaying elective surgical procedures until HbA1c levels are under better control.

5.2 Adrenal disorders

The adrenal glands are small triangular glands located on the superior pole of the kidneys that secrete several hormones that influence wound healing. The cortex of the gland produces corticosteroids (e.g., cortisol), mineralocorticoids (e.g., aldosterone), and androgens. The adrenal hormones are responsible for multiple organ and metabolic functions, including blood glucose regulation, fluid and electrolyte balance, maintenance of blood pressure, and control of the physiologic response to stress. These hormones are critical for maintaining body homeostasis, and severe adrenal insufficiency can be life-threatening.

Failure of the adrenal glands to produce hormones is termed *adrenal insufficiency*. Primary adrenal insufficiency, known as *Addison disease*, is caused by progressive destruction of the adrenal cortices and can occur in the context of autoimmune disease (e.g., systemic lupus erythematosus) or granulomatous disease (e.g., sarcoidosis). The most common findings in Addison disease are weakness, fatigue, hypotension, weight loss, anorexia, nausea, vomiting, and abdominal pain. Abnormal pigmentation of the skin and mucous membranes may develop due to an increased production of adrenocorticotropic hormone (ACTH), which stimulates melanin production via melanocyte-stimulating hormone. Secondary adrenal insufficiency can result from pituitary tumors that interfere with ACTH production, long-term administration of exogenous corticosteroids, or surgical removal of the pituitary gland. Signs and symptoms are often less evident than with primary adrenal insufficiency because aldosterone production is usually normal.

Adrenal crisis is a life-threatening condition that can occur when a patient with adrenal insufficiency (usually primary) encounters stress and cannot produce adequate cortisol and aldosterone to withstand the stressful situation. This results in profuse sweating, dehydration, hypotension, and nausea and requires emergent medical intervention with intravenous corticosteroid administration and fluid and electrolyte replacement to prevent life-threatening severe hypotension, hypothermia, shock, and circulatory collapse.

Excessive levels of cortisol can result from hyperactivity of the adrenal glands (e.g., due to a neoplasm) or more commonly iatrogenically secondary to exogenous corticosteroid therapy. Corticosteroids are metabolized and inactivated by the liver; therefore, patients with compromised hepatic function (see chapter 2) may have prolonged and/or increased effects of corticosteroid therapy. Long-term excessive cortisol levels inhibit white blood cell chemotaxis, leading to chronic immunosuppression, which can compromise wound healing. Moreover, long-term corticosteroid therapy may increase circulating glucose levels, and in diabetics this may further compromise healing capacity due to the effects of prolonged hyperglycemia (section 5.1). *Cushing syndrome* is the clinical term describing the physiologic effects of long-term excess circulating corticosteroids and is characterized by moon faces, weight gain, capillary fragility and bruising, hypertension, and osteoporosis.

5.2.1   *Tests of adrenal function*

Testing for adrenal function is not routine and is not generally ordered in the dental setting. These tests are useful for diagnostic work-up and/or monitoring of patients with known adrenal disorders. Careful assessment of individual patient risk and consideration for ordering of adrenal testing should be done in close collaboration with a physician.

5.2.1.1   *Cortisol*

Cortisol is the primary corticosteroid produced in the cortex of the adrenal glands in response to stimulation by ACTH, which is secreted by the pituitary gland. The production of cortisol follows a circadian pattern, with two-thirds of daily cortisol secreted in the morning hours, and a total daily output of 20–30 mg. This pattern is affected by diet and sleep schedule, such that individuals who sleep during the day and work overnight will have the majority of daily cortisol secretion during the night hours. Physiologic or emotional stress may cause an increased secretion of ACTH and cortisol.

Cortisol levels are not routinely ordered unless the patient has a diagnosed adrenal disorder, or in some circumstances when a patient is taking or has recently discontinued chronic corticosteroid therapy. Patients suspected of having adrenal dysfunction should be referred

Table 5.3 Cortisol equivalent of corticosteroid medications.

Medication	Potency equivalent to cortisol (medication: cortisol)	Medication dose (equivalent to 25 mg of cortisol*)
Hydrocortisone	1:0.8	31.25 mg
Prednisone/Prednisolone	1:4	6.25 mg
Dexamethasone	1:25	0.75 mg

*Approximately the normal daily production of cortisol.

to a physician for further evaluation. Morning serum cortisol levels range between 5 and 20 mcg/dL. Elevated cortisol levels can occur with adrenal tumors, acute (e.g., surgery, trauma, shock, and anxiety) and prolonged stress, chronic high-dose exogenous corticosteroid therapy, and chronic renal failure. Low levels of cortisol may be observed in Addison disease, hepatic disorders, and nephrotic syndrome (renal glomerular dysfunction).

5.2.1.2 *Aldosterone*
Aldosterone is the main mineralocorticoid hormone, produced in the adrenal cortex, and controls renal absorption of sodium and excretion of potassium. Decreased levels of aldosterone indicate primary or secondary hypoaldosteronism, while increased aldosterone (hyperaldosteronism) may be caused by a primary tumor or secondary to high blood pressure, nephrotic syndrome, or hepatic disorders.

5.2.1.3 *Adrenocorticotropic hormone*
ACTH is a pivotal hormone secreted by the pituitary gland that controls adrenal gland function. ACTH regulates the production of corticosteroids, mineralocorticoids, and an androgen precursor known as dehydroepiandrosterone (DHEA). Consistently elevated ACTH levels (due to pituitary tumors or low production of adrenal hormones) lead to hypertrophy and hyperplasia of the inner zones of the adrenal gland cortex, resulting in an increased production of cortisol.

Testing for ACTH levels is ordered to rule-out endocrine dysfunction, such as alterations of the pituitary gland, Cushing syndrome, and adrenal insufficiency. This test, although complementary to cortisol level testing, is more significant than isolated cortisol measurement, as it provides specific information about the physiology of the hypothalamic-pituitary-adrenal (HPA) axis. The ACTH challenge test assesses adrenal gland function by providing an exogenous dose of the hormone and measuring responsive endogenous cortisol production. Failure to produce adequate cortisol following ACTH challenge indicates loss of glandular parenchyma and function. Testing for ACTH is limited to specialized medical laboratories by physician prescription.

5.2.2 *Implications of abnormal tests on provision of oral care*

Patients on long-term high-dose corticosteroid therapy (i.e., 0.5–1 mg/kg or more per day of prednisone/prednisolone) who are planned to undergo more extensive surgical procedures may be at risk for poor wound healing (Table 5.3). There is no laboratory test available to evaluate this level of risk; rather it is based largely on clinical judgment. Antibiotic coverage similar to the antibiotic paradigm for the diabetic patient (section 5.1.2) should be considered. As with DM, any prior history of previous episodes of poor healing should be taken into consideration when treatment planning.

Table 5.4 Steroid supplementation guidelines prior to dental treatment.[*],[†]

Planned dental treatment*	Daily corticosteroid dosage	
	≤ 25 mg cortisol equivalent/day	> 25 mg cortisol equivalent/day
Non-invasive	No supplementation	No supplementation
Minor surgery with local anesthetic	Take usual steroid dose prior to dental appointment	Take usual steroid dose prior to dental appointment
More invasive surgery with local anesthetic	Take usual steroid dose prior to dental appointment	For moderate surgery, take at least 50 mg of cortisol equivalent the morning of surgery (in addition to usual steroid dose) For major surgery or general anesthesia, consult physician for dose adjustment

*No dental treatment recommended if undiagnosed or uncontrolled adrenal insufficiency. There is minimal clinical evidence to support these guidelines and clinicians should always discuss the potential need for steroid supplementation with the patient's managing physician.
†Modified from Miller CS, Little JW, Falace DA. Supplemental corticosteroids for dental patients with adrenal insufficiency: Reconsideration of the problem. J Am Dent Assoc. 2001;132:1570–1579.

Patients on long-term corticosteroid therapy may require steroid dose supplementation prior to surgical interventions to prevent adrenal crisis. This determination is not typically made based on laboratory testing results but rather takes into account the steroid dose, duration of therapy, and the planned procedure. Non-surgical dental procedures do not require steroid supplementation, regardless of the daily corticosteroid dosage. Suggested guidelines for management of surgical stress for minor dental procedures (e.g., simple extraction, soft tissue biopsy, crown lengthening) and more extensive dental procedures (e.g., surgical extractions, quadrant periodontal surgery) are provided in Table 5.4. There is minimal evidence to support these guidelines, and the extent to which such measures are followed varies widely among dentists and specialists. Major surgical procedures performed under general anesthesia are beyond the scope of this clinical guide.

5.3 Bone metabolism

Bone metabolism is characterized in large part by the activity of osteoblasts, which form new bone, and osteoclasts, which mediate bone resorption. The term "bone turnover" refers to the process of bone remodeling that involves osteoclast-mediated bone resorption and osteoblast-induced bone formation. Abnormalities in bone metabolism can affect its ability to heal following injury. Poor healing of the jaws and the development of jaw osteonecrosis are associated with radiation therapy to the head and neck as well as antiresorptive therapies.

Radiation to the jaw as treatment for head/neck cancer is typically provided in doses ranging from 50 to 70 Gray (Gy) and results in compromised bone vitality (see chapter 10). The irradiated bone becomes hypovascular and fibrotic, making it less able to undergo remodeling and healing, and may result in delayed bone repair and development of osteonecrosis, called *post-radiation osteonecrosis of the jaw* (ONJ, Figures 5.3 and 10.9).

Antiresorptive agents inhibit the action of osteoclasts and prevent bone remodeling. Antiresorptive agents include bisphosphonates (oral and intravenous [IV]) and denosumab (subcutaneous and IV), a receptor activator of nuclear factor kappa-B ligand (RANKL, a potent mediator of bone resorption) inhibitor. High-dose (IV) denosumab has been approved

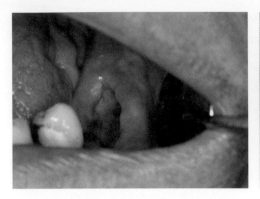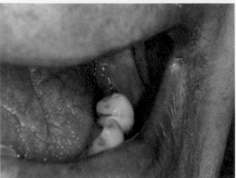

Figure 5.3 Delayed healing of an extraction socket in a patient with a history of radiation therapy for advanced squamous cell carcinoma of the right tonsil.

for the prevention of skeletal-related events from bone metastases in patients diagnosed with solid tumors. Indications for low-dose (oral bisphosphonate and subcutaneous denosumab) antiresorptive therapy include osteopenia and osteoporosis. More intensive high-dose antiresorptive therapy is used in certain cancer patients and is discussed in greater detail in chapter 10. A complication of treatment with antiresorptive agents is the elevated risk for *medication-associated* ONJ. Medication-associated ONJ presents clinically in an identical manner to post-radiation ONJ (see chapter 10).

5.3.1 Bone metabolism tests

5.3.1.1 *C-terminal telopeptide and N-terminal telopeptide*
C-terminal telopeptide (CTX) and N-terminal telopeptide (NTX) assays are indirect measures of active collagen breakdown (type I collagen degradation products, or *pyridynolines*) and osteoclastic activity, and therefore serve as biochemical markers of bone resorption. While these tests cannot be used to make a diagnosis of altered bone metabolism, they may be effectively utilized to monitor bone resorptive activity, for example, to assess risk of fracture in a patient with osteoporosis. In older individuals, particularly in females older than 65 years of age, these markers may be used to evaluate the need for antiresorptive treatment even in the presence of normal bone mineral density findings. A second indication is to monitor response to antiresorptive therapy in cancer treatment. Baseline levels of CTX and NTX are compared to values after 4–6 months of therapy, when maximum antiresorptive activity is reached. There is high variability in these tests related to a variety of systemic factors.

There is no known indication for ordering CTX/NTX tests in dental practice. Antiresorptive agents cause CTX/NTX levels to decrease 40–60% through suppression of bone turnover. This effect may be seen within days in the presence of high-dose antiresorptive therapy, or up to 3 months later for low-dose regimens. It has been suggested that CTX/NTX markers may be utilized to predict an individual patient's risk of developing medication-associated ONJ. However, these markers reflect general skeletal turnover, which does not necessarily correlate with turnover in the maxillofacial region, and the current consensus is that these markers should not be utilized to assess risk of developing ONJ.

5.4   Other considerations

Immune function plays a central role in wound repair by preventing infection and allowing normal healing. Any compromise in the number or function of white blood cells places an individual at greater risk for infection (see chapter 4) and may result in impaired or delayed wound healing. Consequently, in individuals with severely compromised immune systems, antibiotic coverage is recommended on the day of and for 7–10 days following invasive dental procedures. In addition, local wound healing measures such as copious irrigation with saline and placement of sutures in order to obtain primary closure should be considered.

5.5   Suggested literature

Bulger EM, Cuschieri J. Steroids after severe injury: Many unanswered questions. JAMA 2011;305: 1242–1243.

Cremers S, Farooki A. Biochemical markers of bone turnover in osteonecrosis of the jaw in patients with osteoporosis and advanced cancer involving the bone. Ann N Y Acad Sci 2011;1218:80–87.

Farmer A, Fox R. Diagnosis, classification, and treatment of diabetes. BMJ 2011;342:bmj.d3319.

Gibson N, Ferguson JW. Steroid cover for dental patients on long-term steroid medication: Proposed clinical guidelines based upon a critical review of the literature. Br Dent J 2004;197:681–685.

Hoff AO, Toth B, Hu M, Hortobagyi GN, Gagel RF. Epidemiology and risk factors for osteonecrosis of the jaw in cancer patients. Ann N Y Acad Sci 2011;1218:47–54.

Riddle MC, Ambrosius WT, Brillon DJ, Buse JB, Byington RP, Cohen RM, et al. Action to control cardiovascular risk in diabetes investigators. Epidemiologic relationships between A1C and all-cause mortality during a median 3.4-year follow-up of glycemic treatment in the ACCORD trial. Diabetes Care 2010;33:983–990.

Van Poznak CH, Temin S, Yee GC, Janjan NA, Barlow WE, Biermann JS, Bosserman LD, Geoghegan C, Hillner BE, Theriault RL, Zuckerman DS, Von Roenn JH; American Society of Clinical Oncology. American Society of Clinical Oncology executive summary of the clinical practice guideline update on the role of bone-modifying agents in metastatic breast cancer. J Clin Oncol 2011;29:1221–1227.

World Health Organization. Definition and diagnosis of diabetes mellitus and intermediate hyperglycemia. www.who.int, accessed August 1, 2011.

Part B
Guidelines for Diagnosis of Orofacial Conditions

6 Dental Caries and Periodontal Conditions

6.0 INTRODUCTION

Chronic infectious diseases of the oral cavity include dental caries and periodontal diseases. Dental caries causes destruction of the teeth, while periodontal disease is a group of inflammatory conditions that affect the supporting structures of the dentition. The role of the microbial challenge in the initiation and progression of these oral diseases is well established, ultimately leading to the destruction of teeth and/or periodontal structures. This chapter will discuss factors contributing to the diagnosis of dental caries and periodontal diseases.

6.1 Dental caries

Dental caries is a chronic, microbial disease caused by shifts from protective factors favoring tooth remineralization, such as good oral hygiene and fluoride exposure, to destructive factors leading to demineralization, such as plaque formation, frequent ingestion of foods with high carbohydrate contents, and salivary hypofunction. Carious lesions are in a dynamic state of demineralization and remineralization, with fluoride playing an important role in enhancing the remineralization process. Caries results from complex interactions among the tooth structure, the dental biofilm, and dietary, salivary, and genetic influences. *Streptococcus mutans* has been implicated in the etiology of dental caries to cause disease when extracellular polymer formation promotes bacterial attachment and the pH decreases to create a caries-promoting environment. Although *S. mutans* is one of the most researched cariogenic microorganisms, it is only one of more than 500 species found in dental plaque, supporting the hypothesis that *S. mutans* is one of many endogenous microorganisms involved in the complex biofilm that leads to caries activity.

The overall prevalence of dental caries has been declining in the past 40 years, primarily because of increased use of fluoride and more emphasis on oral hygiene, as well as disease prevention and control. Nevertheless, dental caries continues to be a major public health problem, particularly among certain segments of the U.S. population. People of lower socioeconomic status, in particular those who are minorities, homeless, migrants, and children with disabilities, have the highest prevalence and severity of dental caries.

Risk Assessment and Oral Diagnostics in Clinical Dentistry, First Edition.
Dena J. Fischer, Nathaniel S. Treister and Andres Pinto.
© 2013 John Wiley & Sons, Inc. Published 2013 by John Wiley & Sons, Inc.

Table 6.1 Factors contributing to caries risk assessment.*

Caries disease indicators

Clinical	Cavitations into dentin on clinical or radiographic examination White spots on smooth enamel surfaces Restorations placed in the last 3 years due to caries activity
Radiographic	Radiographic enamel interproximal lesions

Caries Risk Factors

Clinical	Deep pits and fissures Root exposure Orthodontic appliances
Behavioral	Visible heavy plaque on teeth Frequent (>3× daily) snacking between meals Diet high in fermentable carbohydrates Recreational drug use
Salivary[†]	Salivary hypofunction (< 1 mg/mL unstimulated) Saliva-reducing factors (medications/radiation/systemic)
Microbiological	Medium or high *Mutans streptococci* and *Lactobacillus* species bacteria counts by culture

Caries Protective Factors

Sealants	Sealants present on permanent molar teeth
Fluoride	Lives/works/school in a fluoridated community Fluoride toothpaste at least once daily
Topical supplements	Fluoride mouth rinse (0.05% NaF) daily 5,000 ppm F fluoride toothpaste daily Fluoride varnish in last 6–12 months[‡] Office fluoride topical in last 6–12 months[‡] Calcium and phosphate supplement paste daily during the last 6–12 months[‡]
Antimicrobial agents	Chlorhexidine prescribed/used daily for 1 week in the last 6–12 months[‡] Xylitol gum/lozenges 4 times daily in the last 6–12 months[‡]
Salivary	Adequate saliva flow (≥ 1 mL/min unstimulated)

*Modified from Dental Clinics of North America, 54(3), Young DA and Featherstone JDB, Implementing caries risk assessment and clinical interventions, pgs. 495–505, 2010 with permission from Elsevier.
[†]See chapter 8.
[‡]Based on routine annual or semi-annual dental visits.

6.1.1   Caries risk assessment

Caries risk assessment (CRA) determines an individual's probability of developing new carious lesions during a specific period of time and the probability of a change in the size or activity of existing lesions over time. This assessment is useful in evaluating the effectiveness of attempts to control caries (e.g., sealants), whether additional diagnostic (e.g., salivary flow rate, diet analysis) and/or caries-control measures (e.g., plaque control, diet control, increased fluoride exposure, antimicrobial agents) are warranted, suitability of treatment plans, and frequency of dental recall appointments.

By assessing patient information, a clinician may be able to predict the risk of future demineralization by weighing all the disease indicators and risk factors against existing protective factors (Table 6.1). *Caries disease indicators* are clinical observations that indicate current caries disease or a history of caries disease. A positive disease indicator automatically places the patient at caries risk. *Caries risk factors* are biologic and behavioral factors that contribute to the level of risk for the patient of having new caries lesions in the future or having existing lesions progress. *Caries protective factors* are biologic and therapeutic factors that may collectively offset the pathologic challenge presented by caries risk factors. With more extensive and severe caries risk factors, the intensity of protective factors must be increased at an appropriate level to minimize the caries process. While there are numerous CRAs available in the literature that similarly measure etiologic and protective factors involved in the disease process, taken together they indicate that past caries experience is the strongest predictor of future caries disease. Examples of CRA tools have been developed and are available through the American Dental Association and American Academy of Pediatric Dentistry.

6.1.1.1   *Caries risk groups*
Implementation of a CRA in clinical practice can be accomplished in a single visit by assessing the CRA components and categorizing a patient as "low," "moderate," or "high" caries risk based upon the prediction of new caries development in the next 1–2 years. Low-risk patients have no active caries, have been caries-free for at least 5 years and have negligble risk factors indicating a very low risk of future dental caries disease. Patients at high risk for caries have active caries status (development of at least one new carious lesion or progression of an existing lesion in the previous 1–2 years), exhibit high-risk behaviors such as frequent ingestion of foods with high carbohydrate contents and poor oral hygiene, and may have additional risk factors such as low to no fluoride exposure and/or salivary hypofunction. Moderate-risk patients have a moderate likelihood of new caries development due to a recent history of caries activity and the presence of risk behaviors and additional risk factors.

Caries management by risk assessment (CAMBRA) is a clinically based approach to preventing, reversing, and, when necessary, repairing early damage to teeth. Clinical intervention protocols vary based upon the caries risk and should be individualized based upon a patient's risk factors and behaviors. Interventions may involve the frequency of bitewing radiographs, frequency of caries recall examinations, choice of restorative materials, and use of salivary tests (flow rate and bacterial culture), antimicrobials (xylitol, a naturally occurring sugar alcohol that maintains the oral pH at 7.0 and inhibits *S. mutans* attachment in the oral environment), fluoride, pH control agents (acid-neutralizing rinses, baking soda gum), calcium phosphate topical supplements, and dental sealants.

6.1.1.2   *Plaque biofilms*
The plaque biofilm is one contributor to the complex caries process, and only biofilm-covered tooth surfaces have the potential to develop carious lesions. Within moments of erupting or being cleaned, tooth surfaces become coated with a protective barrier of molecules (proteins and glycoproteins) derived mainly from saliva, termed the *acquired pellicle*. Bacterial colonizers bind to the acquired pellicle via adhesins and multiply, and as the plaque biofilm develops, the attached bacteria produce extracellular polymers (the plaque matrix) that further consolidate attachment of the biofilm. The microbial composition of the biofilm varies at distinct sites on a tooth and reflects the inherent differences in the anatomy of the tooth and biology of the biofilm. Once established, the composition of the microflora remains stable over time unless there are marked changes to the oral environment. Importantly, the dental plaque bacteria interact and display increased tolerance to both host defenses as well as antimicrobial agents.

6.1.1.3 *Diet*

Dental caries has a strong association with the frequency of fermentable carbohydrate intake. Sticky complex carbohydrates that can remain in the grooves of teeth and simple sugars, particularly sucrose, are very cariogenic. These fermentable carbohydrates are freely diffusible in dental plaque and readily metabolized by oral bacteria, leading to the production of organic acids (e.g., lactic acid) in sufficient concentration to lower the pH of dental plaque enough to allow enamel demineralization to occur. Further, sucrose is involved in the bacterial synthesis of extracellular polysaccharides that can favor the further accumulation of *S. mutans* and other cariogenic bacteria in the dental biofilm. Therefore, reducing the amount and frequency of fermentable carbohydrate consumption is important for people at a high risk of experiencing caries.

6.1.1.4 *Salivary function and buffering capacity*

It is well established that saliva contains numerous protective factors that play a role in maintaining the health of the hard and soft tissues of the oral cavity. Higher salivary flow allows for increased availability of organic and inorganic constituents of saliva, including antimicrobial enzymes and secretory IgA as well as calcium and phosphate ions that maintain the integrity of teeth by regulating the demineralization/remineralization processes. Further, salivary buffering capacity plays a major role in maintaining the oral cavity at a neutral pH, which is optimal for maintaining oral health.

An objective finding of salivary hypofunction (see chapter 8) is a strong indicator of increased caries risk and is an important factor in caries risk assessment, while decreased buffering capacity has a weak but positive association with caries activity. Salivary buffering capacity can be evaluated with chairside commercial kits that assess the bicarbonate buffer system. Dentobuff Strip (Orion Diagnostica, Espoo, Finland) and Saliva-Check Buffer (GC America, Alsip, IL) utilize a few drops of saliva on a test strip and categorize saliva as having poor, intermediate, or normal buffer capacity (see chapter 8). Guidelines regarding the evaluation of salivary buffering capacity in caries risk assessment have not been developed, and the utility of this test remains unclear.

6.1.1.5 *Microbial tests*

Quantification of *S. mutans* and *lactobacilli* in saliva may be utilized to assess caries risk. The theoretical principle behind this test is that high levels of *S. mutans* indicate a cariogenic environment and are associated with an increased caries risk, while high *lactobacilli* counts suggest a high content and frequency of intake of carbohydrates in the diet.

Commercial kits for *mutans streptococci* and *lactobacilli* quantification (CRT bacteria, Ivoclar Vivadent, Amherst, NY; Dentocult SM Strip Mutans and Dentocult LB, Orion Diagnostica, Espoo, Finland; Saliva-Check Mutans, GC America, Alsip, IL) can be performed chairside utilizing saliva or plaque samples (dependent upon the specific kit instructions) on test strips that undergo selective adherence and growth of bacteria. The density of colony growth is evaluated and scored in categories from no detectable growth to high counts (greater than $5–10\times10^6$ colony-forming units). Guidelines regarding microbial quantification in caries risk assessment have not been developed, and the utility of this test remains unclear.

6.1.2 *Diagnosis of dental caries*

Historically, caries was thought to be a progressive disease that eventually destroyed the tooth unless surgical intervention was performed. However, the understanding of the caries process has undergone a paradigm shift. In 2001, a National Institutes of Health Consensus Statement

Table 6.2 Classification of caries lesions in the International Caries Detection Assessment System (ICDAS).*

ICDAS score	Criteria
0	No or slight change in enamel translucency after prolonged air drying (5 seconds)
1	First visual change in enamel (seen only after prolonged air drying or restricted to within the confines of a pit or fissure)
2	Distinct visual change in enamel
3	Localized enamel breakdown in opaque or discolored enamel (without visual signs of dentin involvement)
4	Underlying dark shadow from dentin
5	Distinct cavity with visible dentin
6	Extensive distinct cavity with visible dentin (involving more than half of the surface)

Reprinted from Dental Clinics of North America, 54(3), Braga MM, Mendes FM, and Ekstrand KR, Detection activity assessment and diagnosis of dental caries lesions, pgs. 479–493, 2010 with permission from Elsevier.
*Original table created from data in Ismail AI, Sohn W, Tellez M, Amaya A, Sen A, Hasson H, et al. The International Caries Detection and Assessment System (ICDAS): An integrated system for measuring dental caries. Community Dent Oral Epidemiol 2007;35:170–178.

recommended improved diagnosis of non-cavitated, incipient lesions and non-surgical treatment for prevention and arrest of such lesions. Based on this approach, diagnosis of caries involves establishing the presence or absence of cavitation (*caries lesion detection*) as well as assessing whether or not a lesion is active (*lesion activity assessment*). An active carious lesion progresses over time and requires management (remineralization or restoration), while an inactive lesion may be visible either clinically or radiologically but does not progress or change over time. The combination of lesion detection plus activity assessment is necessary to arrive at the disease diagnosis and the appropriate clinical treatment decisions.

In an attempt to propose an internationally accepted caries detection system, the International Caries Detection Assessment System (ICDAS) was developed by the ICDAS Coordinating Committee (Table 6.2). This system records the status of the surfaces (*unrestored, sealed, restored,* or *crowned*), and then a score is derived based upon the clinical appearance of the carious lesion (visual changes in enamel or dentin). Adjunct criteria have been developed for caries lesion activity assessment and suggest that caries progression is more likely in areas of plaque stagnation and on surfaces that feel rough or soft when a ball-ended probe is gently drawn across the lesion. Nyvad's system is another option for activity assessment of non-cavitated and cavitated caries lesions (Table 6.3). In this system, if the lesion is active and cavitated, treatment is recommended. If active and non-cavitated, non-operative, preventive treatment, such as supplementation with fluoride and remineralization with antimicrobial agents, is recommended. These diagnostic systems are validated caries activity assessment tools that have been used for research purposes and may be utilized in daily clinical practice for detection and assessment of caries activity.

6.1.2.1 *Clinical diagnostic modalities*

Visual detection of dental caries is accomplished after cleaning and drying of teeth. Tactile examination using a dental explorer may also be performed in conjunction with visual examination, though this practice has been considered questionable due to tactile-related surface defects, enlargements, and damage to dental surfaces that may occur. More appropriate strategies involve using explorers to remove plaque and lightly assess surface hardness. Another recommendation is evaluation of the presence of enamel *discontinuities*

Table 6.3 Classification of dental caries.*

Score	Category	Criteria	
0	Sound	Color	– Normal enamel translucency (slight staining allowed in otherwise sound fissure)
		Texture	– Normal enamel texture
1	Active caries (intact surface)	Color	– Enamel surface is whitish/yellowish opaque with loss of luster
		Texture	– Enamel feels rough when tip of probe is moved gently across surface
		Tooth Structure	– No clinically detectable loss of substance
			– Intact fissure morphology; lesion extending along walls of fissure
2	Active caries (surface discontinuity)	Color	– Enamel surface is whitish/yellowish opaque with loss of luster
		Texture	– Enamel feels rough when tip of probe is moved gently across surface
		Tooth Structure	– Localized surface defect (microcavity) in enamel only
			– No undermined enamel or softened floor detectable with explorer
3	Active caries (cavity)	Texture	– Surface of cavity feels soft or leathery on gentle probing
		Tooth Structure	– Enamel/dentin cavity easily visible with naked eye
			– There may or may not be pulpal involvement
4	Inactive caries (intact surface)	Color	– Surface of enamel is whitish, brownish, or black
		Texture	– Enamel may be shiny and feels hard and smooth when tip of probe is moved gently across surface
		Tooth Structure	– No clinically detectable loss of substance
			– Intact fissure morphology; lesion extending along walls of fissure
5	Inactive caries (surface discontinuity)	Color	– Surface of enamel is whitish, brownish, or black
		Texture	– Enamel may be shiny and feels hard and smooth when tip of probe is moved gently across surface
		Tooth Structure	– Localized surface defect (microcavity) in enamel only
			– No undermined enamel or softened floor detectable with explorer
6	Inactive caries (cavity)	Texture	– Surface of cavity feels shiny and feels hard on gentle probing
		Tooth Structure	– Enamel/dentin cavity easily visible with naked eye
			– No pulpal involvement
7	Restoration (sound surface)		
8	Restoration + active caries	Texture	– Caries lesion may be cavitated or non-cavitated
9	Restoration + inactive caries	Texture	– Caries lesion may be cavitated or non-cavitated

Modified from Dental Clinics of North America, 54(3), Braga MM, Mendes FM, and Ekstrand KR, Detection activity assessment and diagnosis of dental caries lesions, pgs. 479–493, 2010 with permission from Elsevier.
*Original table created from data in Nyvad B, Machiulskiene V, Baelum V, Reliability of a new caries diagnostic system differentiating between active and inactive caries lesions. Caries Res 1999;33:252–260.

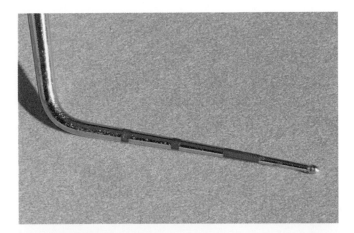

Figure 6.1   World Health Organization periodontal probe.

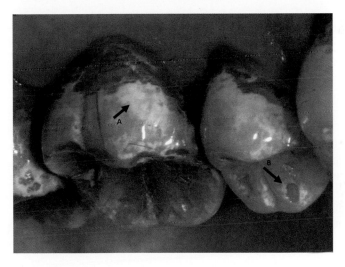

Figure 6.2   Active smooth-surface caries lesions with loss of luster, whitish opaque enamel color, chalky surface texture (A), and localized surface defects (discontinuities, B).

or *microcavitations* using the World Health Organization (WHO) periodontal probe, which is ball-ended with a 0.5 millimeter sphere at the tip (Figure 6.1). When assessing caries lesion activity, active lesions have a softer chalky surface due to increased porosity (Figures 6.2 and 6.3), while arrested lesions have smooth, intact surfaces that reflect light, giving a shiny appearance (Figure 6.3).

6.1.2.2   *Radiographic diagnostic modalities*

Intraoral bitewing radiographs using high-speed film are the conventional method for detecting interproximal caries and are of limited value in detecting occlusal pit-and-fissure or cervical caries. Some disadvantages, however, are that radiographic images underestimate the actual lesion depth and are unable to show accurately the early stages of enamel caries lesions. Decay is difficult to detect in radiographs unless it is greater than 2–3 millimeters deep in dentin or one-third the buccolingual distance. Periapical radiography may be

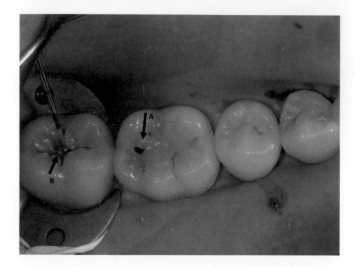

Figure 6.3 (A) Active pit and fissure carious lesion with brownish-black color associated with surface defect and whitish opaque enamel surface with loss of luster; (B) inactive pit and fissure carious lesion with yellowish-brown color as well as smooth, intact surface and shiny appearance.

indicated to assess the proximity of the caries lesion to the pulp and to evaluate periapical tissues and bone loss.

Digital radiography utilizes a digital sensor instead of conventional film and exposes patients to lower radiation doses than conventional methods. Digital images have a diagnostic yield that is equivalent to that obtained by using conventional film, and images can be easily viewed and shared electronically with colleagues. Software programs may be utilized to enhance digital images for more accurate lesion detection. Caries detection software (e.g., Logicon Caries Detector Software, Kodak Dental Systems, Atlanta, GA) has the ability to quantify depth of caries penetration and density. Further, using digital subtraction, two radiographic images of the same site at different time periods can be compared to monitor caries lesion progression.

6.1.2.3 *Classification and quantification of dental caries*
Dental caries can be generally classified based on the location of the lesion. *Pit-and-fissure caries* refers to the development of caries at anatomic landmarks on teeth where the enamel folds inward, most commonly the occlusal (chewing) surfaces of posterior teeth and/or lingual (tongue surface) grooves of maxillary anterior teeth. *Smooth surface caries* occur on the interproximal (surfaces between adjacent teeth), root (portion of the tooth normally covered by gingiva that becomes exposed when gingival recession is present), and/or other smooth surfaces of teeth, particularly the facial/lingual cervical (near the gingiva) surfaces. *Early childhood caries* (ECC) is defined as the presence of one or more decayed (cavitated or non-cavitated) lesions, missing teeth (due to caries), or filled tooth surfaces on any primary tooth in any child 71 months of age or younger (Table 6.4).

Dental caries in an individual can be quantified by calculating the sum of decayed, missing (due to caries), and filled teeth (DMFT) or surfaces (DMFS). These values are calculated for twenty-eight teeth, and a tooth or surface with both caries and a filling is scored as "decayed." Primarily utilized for research and public health surveillance purposes, the

Table 6.4   Definitions of early childhood caries.*

Diagnosis	Definition
Early childhood caries (ECC)	In a child ≤*71 months of age*, ≥1 primary tooth surfaces that are: – decayed (non-cavitated or cavitated) – missing (due to caries) – filled
Severe childhood caries (S-ECC)	In a child *<3 years of age*: – any sign of smooth-surface caries In a child *age 3–5 years*, ≥1 primary maxillary anterior tooth surfaces that are: – cavitated – missing (due to caries) – filled DMFS score of: – ≥4 (age 3) – ≥5 (age 4) – ≥6 (age 5)

DMFS = decayed + missing + filled tooth surfaces
*Table created from data in American Academy of Pediatric Dentistry, American Academy of Pediatrics. Policy on early childhood caries (ECC): Classifications, consequences, and preventive strategies. Pediatr Dent. 2008–2009;30 (7 Suppl):40–43.

DMFT/S can be used to assess prevalence or compare caries status among groups or individuals. One limitation of the DMFT/S is that it does not differentiate between individuals with active caries and those with a past history of caries (i.e., no decayed, only missing and/or filled teeth).

6.1.2.4   *Other diagnostic modalities*

A number of new technologies have been introduced as adjuncts to traditional methods of caries detection. These modalities include the electronic caries monitor, fiber-optic transillumination, and light- and laser-based technologies.

The electronic caries monitor device (ECM, Lode Diagnostic, Groningen, the Netherlands) uses alternating current and measures the bulk resistance of tooth tissue. Porous tissue decreases electrical resistance compared to sound dental tissue, and the ECM is able to detect and quantify this difference. A probe is directly applied to the occlusal surface, and higher numbers indicate deeper caries lesions. This method has not yet been tested on interproximal or facial surfaces and has not received FDA approval as a caries detection device. *Recommendation: ECM performs similarly compared to visual inspection and therefore is of no greater utility than visual inspection for caries diagnosis.*

Fiber-optic transillumination (FOTI) uses a high-intensity white light source to evaluate the relative translucence of a tooth and visualize any discolorations and their extent. Carious enamel and dentin appear as shadows. Digital imaging fiber-optic transillumination (DIFOTI, Electro-Optical Sciences, Irvington, NY) utilizes illumination through a probe that is positioned on the tooth, and then the image is captured digitally and is analyzed with computer software. FOTI and DIFOTI are not able to quantify lesion activity. These devices are FDA approved to aid in the diagnosis of occlusal and interproximal dental caries. *Recommendation: FOTI may serve an adjunctive role with visual inspection to detect early carious lesions.*

Light- and laser-based technologies for caries detection include quantitative light-induced fluorescence (QLF), laser fluorescence, and light-emitting diode (LED) light reflectance and refraction. QLF (Inspektor Pro, Inspektor Dental Care, Amsterdam, the Netherlands) uses a halogen lamp that emits a blue light (370 nm) to fluoresce a tooth. Mineral loss in the tooth causes a decrease in the fluorescence, which appears dark, and the fluorescence is quantified with computer software. Currently, QLF may be utilized to detect progression of demineralization in smooth surface lesions but is unreliable for detecting occlusal and dentin caries lesions. This device is FDA approved to aid in the diagnosis of dental caries. An infrared laser fluorescence device (DIAGNOdent and DIAGNOdent pen, KaVo Dental, Charlotte, NC) emits a red light (665 nm) that is absorbed by bacterial by-products in carious lesions. The resulting fluorescence is quantified; the higher the number, the deeper the caries lesions. The DIAGNOdent pen can be used to assess occlusal and interproximal caries and is FDA approved to aid in the diagnosis of dental caries. LED technology (Midwest Caries I.D., Dentsply Professional, York, PA) analyzes the reflectance and refraction of the LED, which is converted into an electrical signal. The presence of demineralization compared to surrounding tooth structure activates a change in the LED from green to red with a concurrent audible signal. Midwest Caries I.D. has been FDA approved for assessment of occlusal and interproximal caries diagnosis. *Recommendations: QLF may serve an adjunctive role to visual inspection to quantify early mineral changes in smooth surface caries lesions. The DIAGNOdent pen and LED technology may serve adjunctive roles with visual and radiographic methods in detecting occlusal and interproximal lesions.*

Overall recommendation of adjunctive diagnostic modalities for caries detection: While these newer technologies may serve an adjunctive role in caries detection alongside standard visual and radiographic evaluation, they have shortcomings that may not justify routine use in daily clinical practice.

6.2 Periodontal disease

Plaque-induced periodontal diseases have traditionally been divided into three general categories: *health*, *gingivitis*, and *periodontitis*. Health implies that there is an absence of plaque-induced periodontal disease, and the gingiva appears firm and resilient. Gingivitis is a reversible inflammatory reaction of the gingiva to dental plaque biofilms that is characterized by enhanced vascular permeability and influx of inflammatory cells from the peripheral blood into the periodontal connective tissue without loss of connective tissue attachment. Soft tissue alterations include redness, edema, bleeding, and tenderness. Periodontitis is a chronic, non-reversible inflammatory state of supporting tissues around the teeth. The disease begins with colonization and growth of a small group of predominantly Gram-negative anaerobic bacteria and spirochetes, notably *Porphyromonas gingivalis*, *Tannerella forsythensis*, and *Treponema denticola*. *Actinobacillus actinomycetemcomitans* has been observed in aggressive forms of periodontitis. These bacteria extend apically along the tooth roots to induce apical migration of the junctional epithelium, formation of periodontal pockets, and resorption of alveolar bone. If left untreated, the disease continues to progressive bone destruction and ultimately tooth loss. In 1999, the American Academy of Periodontology (AAP) revised the classification of seven major categories of periodontal diseases (Table 6.5). Periodontitis affects approximately 45% of adults in the United States over 50 years of age and is a major cause of tooth mobility and tooth loss worldwide.

Table 6.5   American Academy of Periodontology general categories of plaque-induced periodontal diseases from the International Workshop for Classification of Periodontal Diseases and Conditions.*

Gingivitis

Chronic periodontitis
  – Localized
  – Generalized

Aggressive periodontitis
  – Localized
  – Generalized

Periodontitis as a manifestation of systemic diseases
  – Associated with hematologic disorders
  – Associated with genetic disorders
  – Not otherwise specified

Necrotizing periodontal diseases
  – Necrotizing ulcerative gingivitis
  – Necrotizing ulcerative periodontitis

Abscesses of the periodontium
  – Gingival abscess
  – Periodontal abscess
  – Pericoronal abscess

Periodontitis associated with endodontic lesions
  – Combined periodontic-endodontic lesions

*Table created from data in Armitage GC. Development of a classification system for periodontal diseases and conditions. Ann Periodontol 1999;4:1–6.

6.2.1   Risk factors for periodontal disease

Behavioral risk factors such as oral hygiene compliance and cigarette smoking are well-known preventable risk factors in the development and progression of periodontal disease. Compliance with oral hygiene regimens, particularly plaque control, is a major contributor to the success of periodontal therapy. Cigarette smoking is related to periodontal disease in a dose-related manner, and substances in tobacco smoke may promote the pathogenic activities of periodontal flora. In addition, systemic risk factors such as diabetes mellitus, HIV positivity, host immune response, and stress may contribute to periodontal disease presentation and progression. The relationship between diabetes and periodontal disease is bidirectional, such that patients with poor glycemic control are at risk for more severe periodontal disease, and severe periodontitis may affect the level of glycemic control in diabetic patients. HIV-infected individuals may present with common forms of periodontal disease such as chronic periodontitis and, due to systemic immunocompromise, may also be at risk for necrotizing forms of periodontal disease, which are otherwise rarely encountered in the general population. Consequently, the dental practitioner should encourage risk reduction strategies to improve periodontal prognosis and outcomes.

6.2.1.1   Microbiologic testing for periodontal disease

Microbiologic tests have been developed to identify selected periodontopathic microorganisms in the gingival sulcus. These tests provide information that can potentially guide the clinician in determining whether or not an antimicrobial agent may provide an additional therapeutic benefit for patients who do not respond favorably to mechanical treatment, such as scaling and root planing and periodontal surgical procedures. The AAP Position Paper on Systemic Antibiotics in Periodontics (2004) recommends microbiologic analysis to be performed 1–3 months after completion of mechanical therapy in areas with a poor clinical treatment response to assess the need for antibiotic treatment, followed by re-evaluation with microbiologic testing 1–3 months after antimicrobial therapy. Systemic antibiotic therapy in periodontics should be intense and short term. Subgingival plaque samples are obtained by removing supragingival plaque and then collecting subgingival plaque using curettes or, more commonly, adsorption of microbiologic species onto endodontic paper points. Multiple samples may be obtained from single pockets, or pooled samples (multiple sites per patient) may be utilized to screen patients for the presence of specific bacteria. Commercial oral microbiology testing laboratories provide kits that contain all supplies required for sample collection. For the paper point method of collection, one to two paper points should be inserted to the depth of each periodontal pocket for 10 seconds. Since most periodontal pathogens are highly sensitive to oxygen, specimens should be transferred to transport vials immediately after sampling. The vial cap should not be removed for more than 15–20 seconds to allow for minimal exposure to air. Most oral microbiology laboratories perform sample culturing, which allows for identification and antiobiotic sensitivity analysis of microorganisms, as well as non-culture techniques (which do not require viable cells) including DNA and/or enzymatic activity analysis.

6.2.2   Diagnosis of periodontal disease

Diagnostic parameters that were introduced more than 50 years ago continue to function in clinical practice today. Periodontal disease diagnosis is based on the presence and extent of gingival inflammation, measured as probing depths (PD) of the gingival sulcus, bleeding on probing, clinical attachment loss (CAL), and the pattern and extent of alveolar bone loss assessed radiographically. Conventional diagnostic techniques lack the capacity to identify risk for future periodontal tissue breakdown.

6.2.2.1   *Clinical diagnostic modalities*
PD and CAL evaluation using a periodontal probe (such as the WHO periodontal probe, Figure 6.1) measure damage from past episodes of destruction. Full-mouth examinations at six sites per tooth (mesiobuccal, buccal, distobuccal, mesiolingual, lingual, distolingual) should be performed. PD is the distance from the gingival margin to the base of the gingival sulcus (or "periodontal pocket"), while CAL is the distance from the cementoenamel junction (CEJ) to the base of the sulcus. Generally, increases in PD and CAL of 2–3 millimeters represent disease progression, with CAL being a more accurate measure of disease history and progression than PD. Bleeding on probing is an indicator of gingival inflammation and should be recorded to monitor disease progression or improvement. The location and severity of furcation involvement should be recorded as Class I (beginning), Class II (cul-de-sac), and Class III (through-and-through). Finally, gingival recession, the distance from the CEJ to the gingival margin, and tooth mobility should be noted.

6.2.2.2   *Radiographic diagnostic modalities*
A panoramic radiograph may serve a role in general screening for periodontal disease, though accurate assessment of bone height cannot be ascertained. A full-mouth series of periapical and bitewing radiographs can illustrate the extent and pattern of alveolar bone loss, as well as progression over time, and may be used to measure the severity and extent of periodontal disease. Linear measurements from the CEJ to the alveolar crest and from the CEJ to the base of the osseous defect are commonly used to quantify crestal bone levels and

Table 6.6 Classification of periodontal diseases, modified from the International Workshop for Classification of Periodontal Diseases and Conditions.*

Chronic Periodontitis

Definition		Chronic, non-reversible inflammatory state of supporting tissues around the teeth
Severity	Slight	Loss of ≤ one-third of supporting periodontal tissues Furcation involvement ≤ Class I CAL 1–2 mm PD 3–4 mm
	Moderate	Loss of ≤ one-third of supporting periodontal tissues Furcation involvement ≤ Class I CAL 3–4 mm PD 5–6 mm
	Advanced	Loss of > one-third of supporting periodontal tissues Furcation involvement > Class I CAL > 4 mm PD > 6 mm
Extent	Localized	≤30% of teeth are involved
	Generalized	>30% of teeth are involved

Aggressive Periodontitis

Definition		Rapid attachment loss and bone destruction Patient is clinically healthy, with exception of periodontitis
Severity	Slight	CAL 1–2 mm
	Moderate	CAL 3–4 mm
	Severe	CAL ≥ 5 mm
	Localized	Circumpubertal onset Interproximal attachment loss on ≥2 permanent teeth, one of which is first molar, and involving ≤2 teeth other than first molars and incisors
	Generalized	Patients usually <30 years old Interproximal attachment loss affecting ≥3 permanent teeth other than first molars and incisors

*Table created from data in Armitage GC. Development of a classification system for periodontal diseases and conditions. Ann Periodontol 1999;4:1–6.

osseous defects. Radiographs must show 30–50% demineralization before bone loss can be detected, usually resulting in an underestimation of bone loss. Digital radiography can offer image enhancement and subtraction techniques, which can detect changes in bone density as low as 5% (section 6.1.2.2).

6.2.2.3 *Classification of periodontal diseases*

The AAP utilizes a periodontal disease classification scheme that was developed at the 1999 International Workshop for a Classification of Periodontal Diseases and Conditions (Table 6.6). *Slight* to *moderate chronic periodontitis* involves loss of up to one-third of the supporting periodontal tissues, including Class I furcations. *Slight chronic periodontitis* is defined by CAL of 1–2 millimeters and PD of 3–4 millimeters, while *moderate chronic periodontitis* involves CAL of 3–4 millimeters and PD of 5–6 millimeters. *Advanced chronic periodontitis* is defined as loss of more than one-third of the supporting periodontal tissues with furcation involvement higher than Class I, CAL greater than 4 millimeters, and PD greater than 6 millimeters. Periodontal disease is *localized* if no more than 30% of the teeth are involved, and otherwise it is classified as a *generalized* condition. The AAP has also established case types of periodontitis for the purposes of third-party insurance payments and include *gingivitis* (Case Type I), *mild periodontitis* (Case Type II), *moderate periodontitis* (Case Type III), *advanced periodontitits* (Case Type IV), and *refractory periodontitis* (Case Type V).

Aggressive forms of periodontitis are associated with rapid attachment loss and bone destruction. They are less common than chronic periodontitis and principally affect young patients who are clinically healthy beyond the presence of periodontitis. *Localized aggressive periodontitis* (LAP) is encountered primarily in children and adolescents and is signified by interproximal periodontal destruction of at least two permanent teeth, one of which is the first molar, in the areas of the permanent first molars and incisors. If the destruction occurs around at least three permanent teeth other than first molars and incisors, the diagnosis is *generalized aggressive periodontitis* (GAP), which usually affects patients under 30 years old. Both forms of aggressive periodontitis are plaque-induced infections, but the amounts of microbial deposits are inconsistent with the severity of periodontal tissue destruction.

6.2.2.4   *Other diagnostic modalities*

New diagnostic techniques including biomarkers of disease activity and progression may be utilized in the future to more accurately assess periodontal status and response to treatment. Gingival crevicular fluid (GCF) consituents have been evaluated as potential diagnostic markers of periodontal disease progression. GCF is an inflammatory exudate that can be collected from the gingival sulcus surrounding the teeth and contains inflammatory mediators and tissue-destructive molecules associated with periodontitis. It is in low abundance during health and increases in quantity and complexity of inflammatory molecules with periodontal disease. GCF is collected with methylcellulose filter paper strips placed in the sulci of individual tooth sites, a procedure that can be time-consuming and technique sensitive. Assessment of GCF analytes is laboratory-based; consequently, this biofluid is only used for research purposes at this time.

Two new radiographic technologies may show promise for assessment of small changes in alveolar bone height. Cone-beam computed tomography (CBCT) scans hard tissue structures in a single rotation and creates a three-dimensional image. Local computed tomography (LCT) is a form of CBCT that generates a high-resolution three-dimensional image with dimensions comparable to that of conventional intraoral radiographs. However, these modalities are associated with increased radiation dosage and patient risk compared to conventional radiographic techniques. Another technology, tuned aperture computed tomography (TACT), is a modality that utilizes conventional radiographs taken from different angles that are digitally combined to generate a stack of tomographic slices. LCT as well as TACT and TACT subtraction are developing technologies that may be utilized in the future for detection of osseous changes.

6.3   Selected literature

American Academy of Pediatric Dentistry, American Academy of Pediatrics. Policy on early childhood caries (ECC): Classifications, consequences, and preventive strategies. Pediatr Dent 2008–2009;30 (7 Suppl):40–43.

American Academy of Periodontology. Parameter on chronic periodontitis with advanced loss of periodontal support. J Periodontaol 2000;71(Suppl):856–858.

American Academy of Periodontology. Parameter on chronic periodontitis with slight to moderate loss of periodontal support. J Periodontaol 2000;71(Suppl):853–855.

American Academy of Periodontology Academy Report. Diagnosis of periodontal diseases. J Periodontology 2003;74:1237–1247.

American Academy of Periodontology Position Paper. Systemic Antibiotics in Periodontics. J Periodontology 2004;75:1553–1565.

Armitage GC. Development of a classification system for periodontal diseases and conditions. Ann Periodontol 1999;4:1–6.

Braga MM, Mendes FM, Ekstrand KR. Detection activity assessment and diagnosis of dental caries lesions. Dent Clin N Am 2010;54:479–493.

Ekstrand KR, Martignon S, Ricketts DJ, Qvist V. Detection and activity assessment of primary coronal caries lesions: A methodologic study. Oper Dent 2007;32:225–235.

Fontana M, Zero DT. Assessing patients' caries risk. JADA 2006;137(9):1231–1239.

International Caries Detection and Assessment System Coordinating Committee. Criteria manual for the International Caries Detection and Assessment System (ICDAS II). www.icdas.org, accessed March 30, 2010.

Ismail AI, Sohn W, Tellez M, Amaya A, Sen A, Hasson H, et al. The International Caries Detection and Assessment System (ICDAS): An integrated system for measuring dental caries. Community Dent Oral Epidemiol 2007;35:170–178.

Jenson L, Budenz AW, Featherstone JD, et al. Clinical protocols for caries management by risk assessment. J Calif Dent Assoc 2007;35(10):714–723.

Mol A. Imaging methods in periodontology. Periodontology 2000, 2004;34:34–48.

National Institutes of Health. Diagnosis and management of dental caries throughout life. Consensus Development Conference statement, March 26–28, 2001. J Dent Educ 2001;65:1162–1168.

Nyvad B, Machiulskiene V, Baelum V. Reliability of a new caries diagnostic system differentiating between active and inactive caries lesions. Caries Res 1999;33:252–260.

Young DA, Featherstone JDB. Implementing caries risk assessment and clinical interventions. Dent Clin N Am 2010;54:495–505.

Zero DT, Fontana M, Martinez-Mier EA, Ferreira-Zandona A, Ando M, Gonzalez-Cabezas C, Bayne S. The biology, prevention, diagnosis and treatment of dental caries: Scientific advances in the United Status. JADA 2009;140(9 Suppl):25S–24S.

7 Oral Infection

7.0 INTRODUCTION

Oral infections caused by bacteria, fungi, and viruses are commonly encountered in the general population, and the risk of infection increases dramatically in patients who are immunosuppressed or experiencing salivary gland hypofunction. In the majority of situations, an appropriate clinical diagnosis can be made without the need for laboratory investigation; however, diagnostic testing may be necessary in cases where the clinical presentation of oral infection is abnormal or subdued (which is common in severely immunocompromised patients), or when the diagnosis is known but the infection is non-responsive to standard empirical therapy. Consideration of a patient's risk for infection, as discussed in chapter 4, is an essential component to preventing, diagnosing, and managing patients with oral infections.

7.1 Bacterial infection

Most oral bacterial infections are polymicrobial and of odontogenic etiology and can generally be attributed to an offending tooth and/or supporting structures following clinical and radiographic examination (see chapter 6). Salivary gland and bone infections are far less common but may have a bacterial etiology. Rarely, in the setting of profound and prolonged immunosuppression and/or immunocompromise, non-odontogenic mucosal bacterial infections (e.g., necrotizing stomatitis) may be encountered. In addition, although infrequent, oral bacteria can be isolated during episodes of bacteremia or at distant sites of infection (see chapter 4).

7.1.1 Tests of bacterial infection

Bacterial culturing can be a useful and in some cases critical laboratory test with which all dentists should be familiar (Table 7.1). In the absence of purulence there is no clinical indication for bacterial culturing; results will invariably demonstrate normal oral flora. As most abscesses of odontogenic etiology respond to standard narrow- (e.g., penicillin) or extended- (e.g., amoxicillin) spectrum antibiotics, culturing is generally reserved for cases that are

Risk Assessment and Oral Diagnostics in Clinical Dentistry, First Edition.
Dena J. Fischer, Nathaniel S. Treister and Andres Pinto.
© 2013 John Wiley & Sons, Inc. Published 2013 by John Wiley & Sons, Inc.

Table 7.1 Outline of oral infections, including etiology, clinical presentation, diagnosis, and management.

		Clinical features	Diagnostic tests	Indications for testing	Interpretation of results	Management
Bacterial	Odontogenic	Pain and/or swelling, rarely cellulitis, associated tooth with caries, large existing restoration, or periodontal disease pericoronitis associated with a third molar	Bacterial culture Periapical radiographs or panorex, as indicated	Cultures rarely needed for managing odontogenic infection; indicated when empiric therapy non-responsive with persistent swelling Radiographs indicated in all cases of odontogenic infections	Culture and susceptibility results guide therapy Radiolucent changes associated with apices of teeth generally represent long-standing odontogenic infection	Definitive treatment of associated tooth with endodontic therapy or extraction for pulpal disease, or curettage or extraction for periodontal disease Narrow spectrum antibiotics (penicillin) effective in most infections
	Parotitis	Unilateral painful facial swelling, erythema, pain with eating, purulent (milky) discharge from duct orifice	Bacterial culture Intraoral radiograph, possible CT	Non-response to appropriate empiric therapy; may culture at diagnosis Radiograph may be necessary to evaluate for presence/location of sialolith	Culture and susceptibility results guide therapy, especially when empiric therapy ineffective	Drain purulence via Stensen duct Deliver sialolith (if present) Amoxicillin/clavulanate or other broad-spectrum antibiotic (e.g., clindamycin)
Fungal	Candidiasis	Creamy white plaques throughout oral cavity, erythematous patches, angular cheilitis, burning sensation	Clinical diagnosis primarily—plaques that usually rub off with gauze Fungal culture Cytology	Non-response to appropriate empiric therapy (should fail fluconazole therapy) Atypical clinical presentation when diagnosis is unclear	Culture: Positive culture only diagnostic in context of signs of infection as candida is part of the normal oral flora. Culture may also be utilized to determine susceptibility. Cytology: Presence of characteristic fungal organisms	Topical:Nystatin suspension, swish & spit 1–2 minutes 2–3 times/day Clotrimazole troches, dissolve fully in mouth and swallow 4–6 times/day Systemic: Fluconazole 100–200 mg once daily Ketoconazole 200–400 mg once daily
	Angular cheilitis	Erythema and cracking of the corners of the mouth; may or may not be associated with intraoral candidiasis	Clinical primarily Fungal culture Cytology	Non-response to appropriate empiric therapy; rarely necessary	See "Candidiasis"	Nystatin/triamcinolone cream 2–3 times/day Consider over-the-counter antibacterial ointment (bacitracin/ neomycin/polymixin B) if no improvement after 2 weeks

	Deep fungal	Painful ulcerative/necrotic lesion, most common on palate but can occur in other areas	Biopsy Serology CT/MRI	Non-healing ulcer, in particular in immunocompromised patients Serological tests available for some infections; should only be ordered by infectious disease specialists Imaging studies to assess the extent of disease	Diagnostic histopathologic changes supported by immunostaining for specific organisms	Requires specialized management; may include surgery in combination with intensive long-term antifungal therapy
Viral	HSV	Herpes labialis, crop-like vesicles/ulcerations of the keratinized mucosa, very painful, prodrome common Primary: Primary herpetic gingivostomatitis Secondary: Perioral crusted blistering lesions (herpes labialis, "cold sores" or "fever blisters") Intraoral irregular shallow ulcers affecting the keratinized mucosa In immunocompromised patients can be extensive and affect both keratinized and non-keratinized mucosa	Clinical primarily Viral culture Cytology Direct fluorescence assay (DFA) Serology Biopsy	Atypical presentation Confirmatory diagnosis	Viral culture: Considered the gold standard for diagnosis; however, false negatives may occur Viral cytology: Positive cytologic findings confirm the diagnosis, but unable to type the virus. False negatives can occur if insufficient or non-representative sample collected DFA: Confirmatory typing of a positive culture. This test is often run automatically following a positive culture Serology: Negative HSV IgM and IgG in the setting of acute onset of oral ulcers helps support a diagnosis of primary HSV	Primary: Acyclovir 200 mg 5 times/day for 7 days Valacyclovir 2 g once daily for 7 days Supportive care including pain control, nutritional support and adequate hydration Secondary: Same as primary regimen, need to begin treatment at the earliest onset of prodromal symptoms Topical acyclovir, penciclovir and docosanol also available but generally less effective than systemic therapies

(Continued)

Table 7.1 (Continued)

Clinical features	Diagnostic tests	Indications for testing	Interpretation of results	Management
			Biopsy demonstrates viral cytopathic changes and can be immunostained to confirm the presence of virus. Indicated in atypical presentations where the diagnosis is otherwise uncertain and definitive diagnosis is essential. Typically only in immunocompromised patients	
VZV	Clinical primarily Culture Cytology DFA Serology Biopsy	Confirmatory Inadequate response to empiric therapy	Culture: Positive findings not specific for VZV/HSV; DFA able to confirm. Culture specimen frequently contaminated by oral bacterial flora overgrowth Cytology: Positive cytology does not differentiate between HSV/VZV Serology: Positive serology only demonstrates prior primary infection Biopsy: Biopsy demonstrates viral cytopathic changes and can be immunostained to confirm the presence of virus. Similar to HSV, biopsy only very rarely.	Acyclovir 800 mg 5 times/day for 7–10 days Valacyclovir 1,000 mg 3 times/day for 7–10 days Famciclovir 500 mg 3 times/day for 7–10 days
Primary: Varicella or "chicken pox," may present with oral ulcers **Secondary:** Herpes zoster or "shingles," unilateral intraoral ulcers identical to those caused by HSV, when cranial nerve V involved, facial skin lesions also typical				
CMV	Biopsy	Immunocompromised patients with non-healing oral ulcers	Characteristic histopathologic findings, confirmed by immunohistochemistry	Ganciclovir 1 g 3 times a day until healed Valganciclovir 900 mg twice a day until healed
Oral ulcers, typically solitary and deep, in immunocompromised patients				

EBV	Oral hairy leukoplakia (OHL) Other conditions with orofacial significance: nasopharyngeal carcinoma, Burkitt lymphoma, infectious mononucleosis, post-transplant lymphoproliferative disease	Biopsy (OHL)	Persistent white plaques of the lateral tongue, in particular in a patient with unknown HIV status, especially those at high risk for HIV infection	Characteristic viral cytopathic changes, acanthosis and hyperkeratosis; confirmed by immunohistochemistry	No specific treatment necessary; may respond to systemic acyclovir or valacyclovir therapy A diagnosis of OHL should prompt HIV testing in patients with unknown status
HPV	Benign epithelial proliferations Squamous cell carcinoma of the oropharynx	Biopsy	Excision is definitive treatment for benign lesions Biopsy necessary for suspected squamous cell carcinoma N/A	Distinct and diagnostic histopathologic findings; in cases of malignancy, HPV testing/typing may provide prognostic information	Benign lesions are managed surgically SSC management depends primarily on tumor stage
Enterovirus	Multiple aphthous-like ulcers, soft palate primarily	Clinical only	N/A	N/A	Supportive care only, self-limited infection

CT = computed tomography.
MRI = magnetic resonance imaging.
N/A = not applicable.

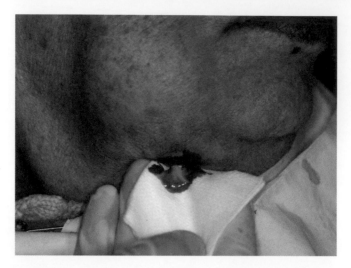

Figure 7.1 This patient with antiresorptive medication-associated jaw osteonecrosis developed a large abscess that was non-responsive to empiric antibiotic therapy. For aerobic culture, the purulent discharge is directly swabbed; however, for anaerobic culture, purulent material should be collected from within the abscess minimizing exposure to air.

non-responsive after at least 48 hours of empiric therapy, so that antibiotic susceptibility testing can be performed. Both aerobic and anaerobic cultures should be collected, and antibiotic susceptibility testing should be requested. For aerobic culture, purulence is sampled directly with a sterile swab and placed with the tip forward into the culture tube and sealed. Anaerobic culture samples for facultative anaerobes should be immediately transferred to transport vials, while strict anaerobe culturing may require a needle aspirate to minimize exposure to oxygen (Figure 7.1). Reporting of results will vary based upon standards at individual laboratories. Non-specific bacterial growth may simply be reported as "normal oral flora," and if abnormal growth is noted, specific organisms are listed. The presence or absence of anaerobes is specified when an anaerobic sample is submitted. Despite optimal technique, it must be recognized that some species are more likely than others to be isolated and identified from clinical specimens; therefore, culture and antimicrobial susceptibility testing results must always be critically interpreted.

Other oral infections that may result in purulence include bacterial parotitis, osteomyelitis, and secondary soft tissue infections associated with osteonecrosis (see chapters 5 and 10). While extremely rare, tuberculosis can manifest with secondary oral lesions that typically present as non-specific ulcerations of the tongue and require incisional biopsy for diagnosis.

7.1.2 Antimicrobials and spectrum

Antimicrobial therapy, whether empiric or based on laboratory results, should always be prescribed according to established or conventional regimens and taken compliantly by the patient for the prescribed duration (Table 7.2). Prescribing the correct antibiotic dose and for an adequate duration is as important as selecting an appropriate antibiotic. Narrow-spectrum antibiotics should be utilized as first-line empiric therapy since these agents are generally efficacious in treating the majority of odontogenic infections.

Table 7.2 Antibiotics commonly used in the management of odontogenic infections.

Antibiotic	Class, mechanism	Spectrum, clinical indication	Regimen
Penicillin	Beta-lactam; bactericidal	Narrow, Gram-positive, first-line for most odontogenic infections	500 mg 4 times a day
Amoxicillin	Beta-lactam; bactericidal	Moderate-spectrum, Gram-positive and some Gram-negative, effective for most odontogenic infections	500–1,000 mg 3 times a day
Amoxicillin/ clavulanate (Augmentin)	Beta-lactam (amoxicillin), beta-lactamase inhibitor (clavulanate); bactericidal	Beta-lactamase resistant, broad-spectrum, Gram-positive/-negative, effective for most severe odontogenic infections	500/125–875/125 mg twice a day
Metronidazole (Flagyl)	Nitroimidazole; selectively targets anaerobes	Anaerobic bacteria, periodontal abscess, in combination with amoxicillin/clavulanate for NUG	250–500 mg 3 times/day
Tetracycline	Tetracycline; bacteriostatic	Broad-spectrum Gram-positive/-negative, not used often for odontogenic infections due to drug resistance	500 mg twice a day to 4 times/day
Doxycycline	Tetracycline; bacteriostatic	Broad-spectrum Gram-positive/-negative Periodontal infection	100 mg twice a day (infection) 20 mg twice a day up to 9 months (periodontitis)
Clindamycin	Lincosamide; bacteriostatic	Aerobic Gram-positive, anaerobic Gram-negative, penicillin allergy	300–600 mg every 6 hours
Cephalexin	Cephalosporin (beta-lactam subcategory); bactericidal	Broad-spectrum, cellulitis	500 mg twice a day
Azithromycin	Macrolide; bacteriostatic	Gram-positive, penicillin allergy, wider spectrum than penicillin	500 mg once a day
Clarithromycin	Macrolide; bacteriostatic	Gram-positive, penicillin allergy, wider spectrum than penicillin	500 mg twice a day

7.1.2.1 *Topical therapy*

Topical antimicrobial therapy can be an important adjunct for management of periodontal disease and secondary soft tissue infection, such as that commonly seen in cases of jaw osteonecrosis. Chlorhexidine gluconate used as a 0.12% topical solution is rinsed for up to 1 minute, twice daily. Chlorhexidine rinses have not been shown to reduce rates of caries or calculus formation, and abscesses require systemic antibiotics with or without surgical intervention.

7.1.2.2 *Systemic therapy*

In general, for any given infection, the most targeted antibiotic with the narrowest spectrum of activity should be utilized. Antibiotics can be bacteriostatic or bacteriocidal, and it is generally best to avoid using combinations of both types of agents concurrently due to potentially competitive mechanisms (Table 7.2). For most odontogenic infections, penicillin

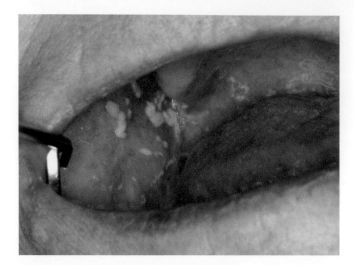

Figure 7.2 Pseudomembranous candidiasis of the buccal mucosa and soft palate in a patient on topical steroid therapy for management of oral lichen planus. Some of the white/yellow plaques are more confluent than others.

is effective, and in the case of a penicillin allergy, clindamycin can be used. For acute suppurative parotitis, a broader-spectrum antibiotic such as amoxicillin, amoxicillin/clavulanic acid, or clindamycin should be considered.

7.2 Fungal infection

Nearly all oral fungal infections are caused by *Candida albicans* or other *Candida* species, which are considered to be normal components of the oral microflora. When the highly balanced oral microbiologic ecosystem is disturbed--for example, due to a shift in the oral bacteria secondary to treatment with antibiotics, or with long-term topical/inhaled corticosteroid therapy--fungal overgrowth and colonization of the mucosa may occur. The most common clinical presentation of a fungal infection in the mouth is *pseudomembranous candidiasis*, characterized by multiple white or yellow papules that colonize the oral soft tissues, appearing similar in consistency to cottage cheese and usually can be scraped off or removed with gauze (Figure 7.2). *Erythematous* (or *atrophic*) *candidiasis*, presenting as an area of mucosal redness, is less common than the pseudomembanous form but must be considered in patients with symptoms of oral burning/discomfort, especially those with salivary gland hypofunction and/or use of a dental prosthesis (Figure 7.3). *Chronic hyperplastic candidiasis* is rare and presents clinically as an area of leukoplakia and/or hyperplastic tissue. Due to the clinical presentation, biopsy is typically necessary for diagnosis, and systemic therapy is required for management. *Angular cheilitis* is most commonly caused by superficial fungal infection and is characterized by raw, erythematous lesions at the lip commissures (Figure 7.4).

Deep fungal infections (e.g., aspergillosis, cryptococcosis, blastomycosis, histoplasmosis, paracoccidioidomycosis, and mucormycosis) of the oral cavity are very rare and are almost exclusively encountered in immunocompromised individuals. These infections typically present as ulcerative lesions and require biopsy for diagnosis. Since oral lesions are usually associated with primary infection of the respiratory tract (e.g., sinuses, lungs), imaging studies are also included as part of the diagnostic work-up.

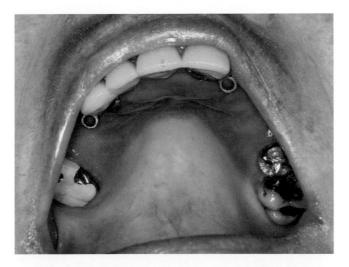

Figure 7.3   Erythematous candidiasis of the palate following the precise outline of the patient's acrylic-based removable partial denture.

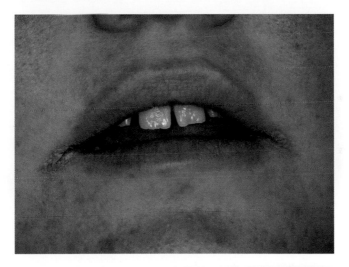

Figure 7.4   Angular cheilitis in a patient with Crohn disease with erythema and cracking of the corners of the mouth.

7.2.1   Tests of fungal infection

An astute clinician should usually be able to make the diagnosis of candidiasis by history and physical exam alone, without the need for laboratory testing. As *Candida* species are normal components of the oral flora, fungal culture, even in the absence of overt clinical signs of infection, will often be positive. Given that both topical and systemic antifungal therapies are generally safe and highly effective, empirical therapy should be prescribed following a provisional clinical diagnosis (Table 7.3). Similar to the use of bacterial culturing, fungal culture should be reserved for only those cases that do not initially respond to appropriate antifungal therapy. Utilizing the same kit used for aerobic bacterial culturing,

Table 7.3 Antifungal regimens for the management of oral candidiasis.

Antifungal agent	Class	How supplied	Dispensation instructions	Regimen	Notes
Topical					
Nystatin	Polyene	100,000 units/mL suspension	One bottle (473 mL)	Swish and spit (or swallow if esophageal lesions) for 1–2 minutes 2–3 times/day; continue until lesions resolved	Efficacy varies; if lesions do not respond, treat with systemic agent
Clotrimazole	Azole	10 mg troche	One bottle (70 or 140 troches)	Let one troche dissolve fully in the mouth, 4 times/day	Troches will not dissolve in patients with significant dry mouth
Nystatin/triamcinolone acetonide	Polyene and corticosteroid	Cream	One tube (15 g, 30 g, or 60 g)	Apply a small amount to the corners of the mouth twice daily for *angular cheilitis*	Signs and symptoms generally respond within 2–3 days
Systemic					
Fluconazole	Azole	Tablet (100 mg, 150 mg, 200 mg) Oral suspension (40 mg/mL)	One-month supply (30 tablets). While a full 30-day regimen is rarely required, this ensures sufficient medication in the event of recurrence or difficult-to-treat cases.	Take one tablet once daily; a 7-day course is generally sufficient for complete resolution of candidiasis. In patients with recurrent infection treatment with one 100 mg tablet once or twice weekly is in most cases highly effective.	True resistance to fluconazole is rare; in the event of poor response, culture with sensitivity testing and empirically increase dose (e.g., from 100 mg to 200 mg) Oral suspension is useful for patients with difficulty swallowing pills. There is no evidence that *topical* fluconazole is any more effective than nystatin or clotrimazole

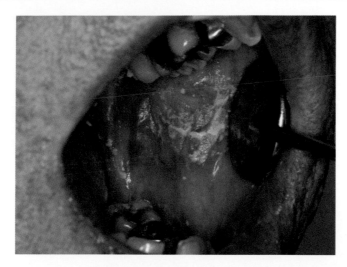

Figure 7.5 Persistent erythematous and pseudomembranous candidiasis despite high-dose fluconazole therapy in a patient on long-term immunosuppressive therapy. Culture and sensitivity demonstrated fluconazole resistance but voriconazole susceptibility.

the affected area (pseudomembrane or erythema) is swabbed and transported to the laboratory in the same manner. In such cases, both culture and sensitivity (antimicrobial susceptibility) testing should be ordered to guide effective therapy (Figure 7.5, Table 7.1).

Exfoliative cytology is a test that can confirm the diagnosis of candidiasis. Suspected fungal infections are scraped with a wood spatula to obtain cellular material that is smeared on a glass slide and treated with a fixative, then packaged and sent to a pathology lab for cytopathologic evaluation. At the laboratory, the slide is treated with potassium hydroxide (KOH), lactophenol blue or other dye, or fixed and stained with periodic acid-Schiff (PAS), and evaluated microscopically for the presence of characteristic fungal organisms (see chapter 1, Figure 1.9). Cytology specimens can determine the presence or absence of yeast but cannot be evaluated for fungal species or antifungal susceptibility testing.

Tissue biopsies can be stained with PAS to identify the presence of invasive fungal hyphae within the epithelium (Figure 7.6). Positive findings must be interpreted carefully in the absence of clinical signs of infection. In the case of a suspected deep/invasive fungal infection, a positive biopsy specimen will demonstrate characteristic features that can be further confirmed with a series of immunohistochemical stains. Further work-up for a suspected deep fungal infection should be coordinated by an infectious disease physician and may include imaging studies (plain film or CT of the chest, sinuses, or other areas of suspected disease), serologic tests (mannan and galactomannan antigen tests), and/or bronchoalveolar lavage.

7.3   Viral infection

Viral infections that may affect the oral cavity include members of the human herpes virus family (herpes simplex 1 and 2, varicella zoster virus, cytomegalovirus, and Epstein-Barr virus), human papillomaviruses, and enteroviruses. Oral viral infections present with a wide variety of clinical features, ranging from painful ulcerations to asymptomatic exophytic papillary soft tissue lesions, with management being dependent upon accurate diagnosis.

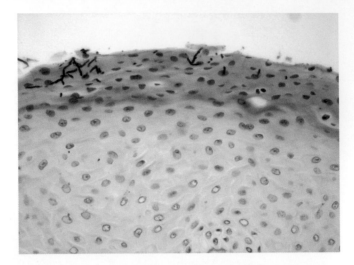

Figure 7.6   Biopsy specimen of an erythematous tongue lesion from the same patient in Figure 7.5 following voriconazole therapy. Despite apparent clinical resolution of candidiasis, the PAS stain demonstrated evidence of continued fungal infection (filamentous rods in keratinized epithelium).

Oral aphthous ulcerations (see chapter 11) are commonly attributed to "viral" infection but are not infectious in etiology. The one viral condition that can mimic aphthous ulceration is *herpangina* (enterovirus infection), which is characterized by multiple aphthous-like ulcers that are generally restricted to the soft palate. The clinical features, diagnosis, and management of the most commonly encountered viral infections of the orofacial region are summarized in Table 7.1.

7.3.1   Tests of viral infection

Tests used for the diagnosis of oral viral infections and viral-mediated lesions include culture, cytology, biopsy, and serology (Table 7.1). Appropriate use of these tests, along with a proper history and examination, may be necessary to determine the correct diagnosis and guide effective therapy. Patients with signs/symptoms of herpes simplex virus (HSV) infection should be treated empirically even when diagnostic tests are utilized so as to avoid any delays in providing effective management and relief of symptoms. Rather than including a discussion of all diagnostic tests that can be used to evaluate viral infection (including, e.g., lumbar puncture), this chapter emphasizes only those tests that may be of practical clinical utility for oral health care practitioners.

7.3.2   Viral culture

Viral culturing is a technique-sensitive investigation that requires careful coordination with the analyzing laboratory due to the temperature-sensitive nature of the virus; for this reason, viral culture is typically limited to practices with an on-site laboratory or regular pick-up service. Ulcerative lesions are lightly swabbed with the sterile tip, which is then placed tip down into the liquid medium and sealed; crusted lesions must be "unroofed" in order to obtain an adequate sample (Figure 7.7). The specimen is placed in viral culture transport medium and transported immediately after collection or maintained on ice when using an

(a)

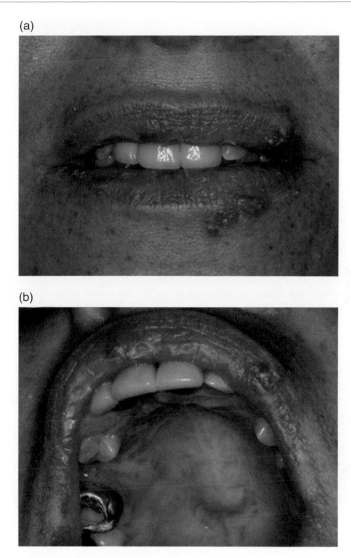

(b)

Figure 7.7 Recrudescent HSV infection in an immunocompromised patient presenting with intact vesicles of the lips (a) and multiple shallow crop-like ulcerations of the hard palate (b). The intraoral lesions could be swabbed; however, the lip lesions would need to first be unroofed in order to obtain an adequate culture sample.

off-site laboratory. Positive results can be obtained in as little as 24–48 hours; however, in some cases definitive results may take 7–10 days. Importantly, HSV culture has very high specificity but low sensitivity (~50%); therefore, culture results may be negative even in the presence of what appears to be obvious infection.

Direct fluorescence antibody (DFA) *test* is a rapid diagnostic HSV test that is useful when a confirmatory and specific (e.g., HSV-1, HSV-2, VZV) diagnosis is required. DFA is typically ordered following a positive viral culture result to confirm virus typing. *Polymerase chain reaction* (PCR) is an extremely sensitive assay that is used primarily for testing of cerebrospinal fluid and is rarely utilized for evaluating oral lesions; however, tests are available for most of the human herpes viruses.

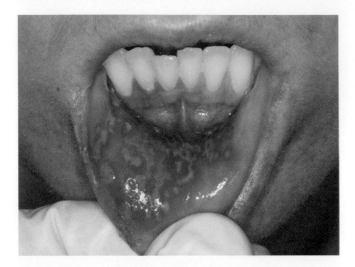

Figure 7.8 Primary HSV infection that was initially believed to be recurrent herpes zoster infection due to the primarily unilateral distribution of lesions. Serology did not demonstrate anti-HSV IgM or IgG and viral culture confirmed HSV-1 positivity.

7.3.3 Viral cytology

Similar to the use of cytology for evaluating fungal infections, viral cytopathology provides diagnostic results in a minimally invasive manner. Positive cytologic smears for herpes virus infection demonstrate typical virally induced cellular changes that include multinucleated giant cells and "ballooning" degeneration of the nucleus in the cytoplasm (see chapter 1, Figure 1.8). Viral cytology is useful when an immediate diagnosis is required, culture results are inconclusive, and/or empiric therapy is ineffective. However, while viral cytology can determine the presence or absence of virus, a specific diagnosis (e.g., HSV) cannot be made from cytology results alone. As is the case with culture, an adequate sample must be obtained, and any crusting must be removed in order to obtain proper cellular material from the ulcer base (see chapter 1). For these reasons, obtaining a viral cytologic sample can be associated with significant patient discomfort.

7.3.4 Viral serology

Serologic tests for presence of viral antibodies as well as quantitative measurement of virus are used extensively in medicine. However, for the purposes of evaluating patients with oral infections, serologic tests are rarely necessary. Positive serology for HSV IgM antibodies (at least four-fold increase) signifies primary or acute HSV infection and may be of some use in atypical cases where the diagnosis is unclear. The presence of IgG antibodies only confirms prior exposure but may be useful to determine whether or not a patient was previously infected (Figure 7.8). As serologic testing results are not immediate, empiric therapy should be initiated when there is strong clinical suspicion for viral infection.

7.3.5 Biopsy

In some cases, tissue biopsy is necessary to determine the correct diagnosis of viral lesions. Any lesions of unclear etiology that do not respond to appropriate empiric therapy and cannot be diagnosed by other means require biopsy.

7.4   Factors that may contribute to infection

A number of factors can affect an individual's risk of developing an oral infection. The two most important factors are immune status and salivary gland function, both of which are covered in much greater detail in chapters 4 and 8.

7.4.1   Immunosuppression

The immune system plays a central role in both the prevention and resolution of oral infections. The two most important factors are the degree and duration of immunosuppression. Immunosuppression can develop secondary to underlying systemic disease, as is the case with AIDS and acute leukemias, or much more commonly secondary to medical treatment, including cancer chemotherapy and the use of immunosuppressive and immunomodulatory therapies. The most commonly encountered oral infections linked to decreased immune function are oral candidiasis and recrudescent HSV. With increased degree of immunosuppression, not only is the risk of developing infection increased but the response to treatment may be reduced, requiring an extended and more intensive course of therapy.

7.4.2   Salivary gland hypofunction

Saliva plays a multitude of critical roles in maintaining physiologic equilibrium in the oral cavity. With respect to oral infections, saliva serves a protective role in minimizing the initiation and progression of dental caries and suppressing superficial fungal colonization of the oral mucosa. When this balance is altered, due to quantitative and/or qualitative changes in saliva, the risk of infection is greatly increased. The impact of additional risk factors for dental caries (e.g., poor oral hygiene, high carbohydrate diet) and candidiasis (e.g., use of topical steroids) is further exacerbated in the presence of salivary gland hypofunction.

7.5   Selected literature

Gafter-Gvili A, Fraser A, Paul M, et al. Meta-analysis: Antibiotic prophylaxis reduces mortality in neutropenic patients. Ann Intern Med 2005;142(12 Pt 1):979–995.

Lerman MA, Laudenbach J, Marty FM, et al. Management of oral infections in cancer patients. Dent Clin North Am 2008;52(1):129–153.

Levi ME, Eusterman VD. Oral infections and antibiotic therapy. Otolaryngol Clin North Am 2011;44(1): 57–78.

Saral R, Burns WH, Prentice HG. Herpes virus infections: Clinical manifestations and therapeutic strategies in immunocompromised patients. Clin Haematol 1984;13(3):645–660.

8 Salivary Conditions

8.0 INTRODUCTION

Saliva is essential for normal oral function and homeostasis. Salivary flow from the paired major (parotid, submandibular, and sublingual) and numerous minor salivary glands is controlled by the sympathetic nervous system. Functionally, saliva moistens and lubricates the surface of the tongue and other hard and soft tissues during mastication and swallowing. Immunologically, saliva plays an essential role in the control of oral infections (see chapter 7), by the actions of salivary components that include secretory IgA (sIgA), lactoferrin, lysozyme, and histatin. Saliva also has anti-caries properties (see chapter 6) demonstrated by (a) its antibacterial properties mediated through antimicrobial enzymes and sIgA; (b) its buffering capacity, which maintains a neutral pH environment; and (c) its important role in enamel remineralization by continuously bathing the teeth in calcium and phosphate ions that are reincorporated into the enamel matrix.

Any compromise in saliva production or quality can result in significant short- and long-term effects on the oral mucosa, dentition, and overall health. These changes may also secondarily alter the oral flora, creating a more "cariogenic" environment. Clinically, patients usually become aware of changes in quality and quantity of saliva when the feeling of oral dryness develops. *Xerostomia*, defined as the patient's report of oral dryness, is a common complaint that may or may not correlate with *salivary hypofunction*, an objective finding of decreased salivary flow. Hydration status has an important impact upon salivary gland hypofunction. Systemic diseases, such as diabetes and autoimmune conditions, as well as use of several medications, have also been associated with salivary gland dysfunction (Table 8.1).

In addition to compromised function, the salivary glands are also subject to infectious, inflammatory, obstructive, and neoplastic conditions. This chapter will review the diagnosis of common salivary gland disorders.

Risk Assessment and Oral Diagnostics in Clinical Dentistry, First Edition.
Dena J. Fischer, Nathaniel S. Treister and Andres Pinto.
© 2013 John Wiley & Sons, Inc. Published 2013 by John Wiley & Sons, Inc.

Table 8.1 Medications associated with xerostomia.

Class	Examples
Antidepressants	Duloxetine (Cymbalta), fluoxetine (Prozac)
Antiemetics	Ondansetron (Zofran), metoclopramide (Reglan)
Antihistamines	Diphenhydramine (Benadryl), fexofenadine (Allegra)
Antihyperlipidemics	Atorvastatin (Lipitor), simvastatin (Zocor)
Antimuscarinics/spasmodics	Tolterodine (Detrol), oxybutynin (Oxytrol)
Antipsychotics	Olanzapine (Zyprexa), lithium carbonate (Eskalith)
Benzodiazepines	Clonazepam (Klonopin), diazepam (Valium)
Diuretics	Bumetanide (Bumex), furosemide (Lasix)
Hypnotics	Eszopiclone (Lunesta), zolpidem (Ambien)
Opioid analgesic combinations	Oxycodone/acetaminophen (Percocet), hydrocodone/acetaminophen (Vicodin)
Muscle relaxants	Tizanidine (Zanaflex), cyclobenzaprine (Flexeril)
Non-steroidal anti-inflammatory drugs	Naproxen (Aleve), etodolac (Lodine)
Proton pump inhibitors	Omeprazole (Prilosec), esomeprazole (Nexium)

8.1 Implications of salivary hypofunction

8.1.1 Local infection

Patients with significant salivary gland hypofunction are at an increased risk for developing recurrent oropharyngeal candidiasis (see chapter 7) and rampant dental caries (see chapters 6 and 10). Candidiasis is frequently encountered in patients with severe salivary hypofunction, and patients with recurrent episodes may require long-term prophylactic therapy. Dental caries present most frequently at gingival margins (where food debris collects) and interproximally. For this reason, bitewing radiographs should be obtained routinely (every 6–12 months) and use of fluoride and remineralizing products should be prescribed in patients with significant salivary hypofunction.

8.1.2 Dysphagia

Decreased salivary flow may result in significant difficulties with chewing and swallowing. The moisturizing and enzymatic functions of saliva are critical for the formation of a soft bolus for deglutition. Copious amounts of fluid may be needed to aid with swallowing so that food does not lodge in the esophagus. Furthermore, patients with severe salivary hypofunction may be at risk for aspiration of food into the larynx, causing an elevated risk of airway obstruction and aspiration pneumonia. Patients with a history of recurrent episodes of dysphagia or esophageal blockage should be referred to a gastroenterologist for further evaluation.

8.1.3 Oral discomfort

Patients with salivary gland hypofunction often describe a generalized sensation of mouth discomfort due to the lack of moisture and lubrication. Persistent dryness may cause mucosal sensitivity to flavored or spicy food and drinks, and in some cases there may be a complaint of a persistent burning sensation in the absence of any recognized cause. This is a clinical

Table 8.2 Medications associated with taste changes.

Class	Examples
ACE inhibitors	Captopril (Captopril), enalapril (Vasotec)
Analgesics	Acetylsalicylic acid (aspirin), nabumetone (Relafen)
Antibiotics	Metronidazole (Flagyl), penicillin V (Veetids)
Anticonvulsants	Carbamazepine (Tegretol), phenytoin (Dilantin)
Antidiabetics	Metformin (Glucophage), glipizide (Glocotrol)
Antigout	Allopurinol (Zyloprim), colchicine (Colcrys)
Antimanics	Lithium carbonate (Lithium), risperidone (Risperdal)
Antimetabolites	Methotrexate (Trexall), hydroxyurea (Hydrea)
Antiparkinsonians	Levodopa (Sinemet), benztropine mesylate (Cogentin)
Antituberculars	Ethambutol (Myambutol), isoniazid (Nydrazid)
Hormone replacements	Thyroxine (Synthroid), estrogen (Premarin)
Proton pump inhibitors	Prilosec (Omeprazole), esomeprazole (Nexium)

symptom that should not be confused with burning mouth syndrome (see chapter 12), a condition that is defined by the absence of any underlying cause or disorder.

8.1.4 *Dysgeusia*

Taste perception is a complex process mediated by sensory input to nerve endings (from cranial nerves VII, IX, and X) located in the oral mucosa, mostly on the dorsal tongue. Saliva plays a key role in transmitting taste signals, and *dysgeusia* (altered taste) or *hypogeusia* (diminished taste) may be reported by patients with low salivary flow. Abnormalities range from decreased or altered perception of certain or all tastes (sour, bitter, salty, sweet) to a complete loss of taste (*ageusia*). The diagnosis of dysgeusia is primarily based on patient history and is discussed in more detail in chapter 10. Importantly, some medications may cause taste abnormalities without directly affecting salivary flow, especially angiotensin-converting enzyme (ACE) inhibitors and hormone replacement therapy (Table 8.2). There is limited effective treatment for dysguesia; patients may benefit from referral to centers that specialize in taste and smell disorders.

8.2 Diagnostic tests for saliva and salivary glands

8.2.1 *Measurement of xerostomia and salivary hypofunction*

Xerostomia is more frequently assessed than salivary gland hypofunction, which requires objective measurement of salivary flow. Subjective and objective measures of mouth dryness are not always well correlated, and it is not uncommon for a patient complaining of xerostomia to have normal salivary flow rates. Numerous studies have demonstrated that assessment of xerostomia is a better reflection of patient symptoms and is a useful guide for management. Several instruments, such as the the *Xerostomia Inventory* and the *Xerostomia Intensity Scale*, measure the severity of mouth and lip dryness and impact on a patient's ability to perform oral functions such as swallowing and speaking. Although these validated scales appear to be useful in assessing xerostomia severity and its impact over time, a significant limitation is the inability to actually diagnose and score xerostomia using these tools.

Unstimulated saliva collection (draining method)	Stimulated saliva collection (draining method)
Supplies	*Supplies*
Distilled water, pre-weighed cups, and scale with accuracy of 0.01 g.	Distilled water, pre-weighed cups, scale with accuracy of 0.01 g, 2% citric acid solution with cotton swabs or gum base. The citric acid solution can be compounded by any pharmacy.
Instructions:	*Instructions:*
The collection period will last 5 minutes.	The collection period will last 5 minutes.
• Have patient rinse his/her mouth with distilled water and relax for five minutes. • With the head leaned forward over the pre-weighed cup, ask the patient to swallow once and then allow saliva to collect *without swallowing* for the next 5 minutes (start timer). • Every minute for the next 5 minutes, ask the patient to spit saliva into the cup. • After 5 minutes, weigh the cup with saliva and subtract the pre-weighed value to obtain the 5-minute whole salivary flow rate. The resulting value in milligrams = equal number of milliliters (gravimetric method).	• Have patient rinse his/her mouth with distilled water and relax for five minutes. • With the head leaned forward over the pre-weighed cup, ask the patient to swallow once and then allow saliva to collect *without swallowing* for the next 5 minutes (start timer). • Flow stimulation: A) Apply (2%) citric acid with cotton swabs on dorsal tongue for 3 seconds, every 30 seconds, or B) Chew gum base. • Every minute for the next five minutes, ask the patient to spit saliva into the cup. • After 5 minutes, weigh the cup with saliva and subtract the pre-weighed value to obtain the 5-minute whole salivary flow rate. The resulting value in milligrams = equal number of milliliters (gravimetric method).

Normal salivary flow rates:

Saliva source	Threshold for hyposalivation
Unstimulated whole saliva	< 0.1 mL/minute
Stimulated whole saliva	< 0.7 mL/ minute

Figure 8.1   Salivary flow collection procedures and measurement protocols.

Objective assessment of salivary flow can be a useful diagnostic tool to validate symptoms of xerostomia and may be included as part of the diagnostic work-up for Sjögren syndrome. Salivary flow measurements may also be used to evaluate response to therapy. Salivary function is assessed by sialometry, in which salivary flow is measured volumetrically over an established period of time and compared to normal values. Salivary flow rates for healthy adults have been normalized using population-based data. Flow measurement can be gland-specific (parotid, submandibular/sublingual) or whole (all glands including minor glands) and can be evaluated at rest (unstimulated) or after stimulation. A normal value for whole unstimulated saliva is a volume greater than 0.1 milliliters (mL) per minute, while that for stimulated saliva is greater than 0.7 mL per minute; gland-specific standard values have not yet been established. Since flow rates may fluctuate with circadian rhythm, collection should be performed in the morning when there is less variability, and consecutive collections in the same patient should always be performed under the same conditions.

The simplest and most frequently used salivary collection technique is the draining method, in which the patient expectorates pooled saliva into a pre-weighed container (Figure 8.1). Additional methods of saliva collection are primarily used for research purposes and include mechanical draining, mechanical suction, and the use of saliva collectors. Mechanical draining is accomplished with an electric laboratory pipette placed in the floor

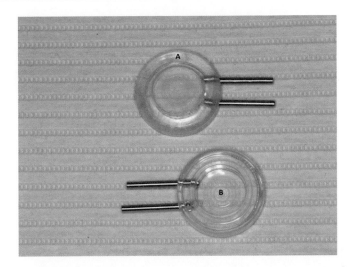

Figure 8.2 Carlson-Crittenden collectors. Saliva drains gravimetrically to the bottom orifice (B) and through the collector to the adjacent tubing. The outer ring (A) is used to establish negative pressure on the buccal mucosa to maintain the collector in place.

of the mouth, removing saliva (combined submandibular/sublingual) when a "pool" of saliva accumulates (salivary pooling). Parotid flow is collected via a mechanical suction device called the Carlson-Crittenden cup, in which the suction device is placed over the Stensen duct orifice (Figure 8.2). Hydroxycellulose sponges and polyester/cortisol rolls can be placed in the mouth to absorb saliva. This method is often used for research purposes to obtain saliva for biochemical or biomarker studies.

8.2.2   Tests of salivary constituents

The use of saliva as a diagnostic fluid has drawn attention in recent years as a simple and non-invasive way to measure serologic markers including multiple electrolytes, hormones, and proteins. A number of commercial tests are now available for various indications ranging from HIV diagnosis to drug monitoring. The utilization of saliva as a diagnostic fluid is addressed in more detail in chapter 2. Salivary tests that assess quality of saliva are described below.

8.2.3   Salivary pH and buffering capacity

The pH of saliva is approximately 7.4 in healthy individuals and serves both as a defense against oral bacteria and as a buffer against enamel demineralization. Decreased salivary pH has been proposed as a risk factor for progression of smooth surface dental caries and enamel erosion. Salivary pH is measured colorimetrically using strips of pH paper (litmus strips, available through dental supply companies) that undergo a change in color, which correlates with the salivary pH. Despite the theoretical association with the risk of dental caries, assessment of salivary pH has not proven to be a reliable test for this purpose and therefore its clinical use is limited.

   The buffering capacity of saliva is the ability of saliva to decrease or neutralize the acids produced by oral bacteria and thereby prevent or reduce dental caries. Buffering is primarily

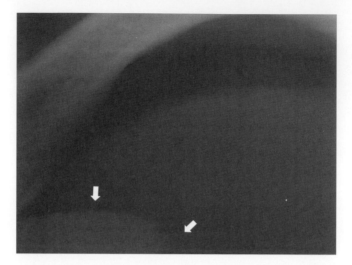

Figure 8.3 Occlusal film demonstrating a right submandibular gland sialolith in an asymptomatic 71-year-old female.

mediated through the carbonic acid/bicarbonate system, and the buffering capacity of an individual's saliva can be measured using commercial kits with test strips (see chapter 6). Guidelines regarding the evaluation of saliva buffering capacity are lacking, therefore the utility of this test in high-risk caries populations is still unclear.

8.2.4 *Imaging studies*

Imaging of the salivary glands is performed when there is suspicion of neoplasm or masses (growth, asymmetry, or change in size), obstruction (stones or strictures), infection, or as part of a series of diagnostic studies to evaluate salivary function. Basic plain film imaging can be performed in the dental setting, while advanced techniques generally require referral to a larger medical center.

8.2.4.1 *Radiography*
Occlusal (plain) films of the floor of the mouth can be used to evaluate stone formation in the submandibular or sublingual gland ducts and present as variable radiopaque structures (Figure 8.3). Sialography may be indicated when there is a suspected obstruction of a major salivary gland or alteration of normal ductal parenchyma, but this test may result in patient discomfort (swelling and tenderness) and is contraindicated in patients sensitive to the imaging dye (see chapter 1).

8.2.4.2 *Ultrasonography*
Ultrasound is useful for detection of superficial masses or cysts. The advantages of ultrasound are that it does not expose the patient to radiation and does not require injection of a contrast agent. However, deep structures cannot be adequately visualized, and images should only be interpreted by radiologists with experience in the evaluation of salivary gland ultrasounds.

8.2.4.3 *Scintigraphy*

Scintigraphy simultaneously evaluates the condition of salivary gland parenchyma and its functional capacity. While assessment of functional capacity is the main advantage of scintigraphy compared to other imaging modalities, there is still no accepted gold standard for quantification of glandular function. Scintigraphy involves the use of ^{99m}Tc-sodium pertechnectate, a radioactively labeled tracer that is taken up by the salivary glands. Uptake at two different time points is measured and compared to assess function. Scintigraphy is only performed at specialized imaging centers, usually within a major hospital center, and its use is largely limited to research.

8.2.4.4 *Magnetic resonance imaging*

MRI of the salivary glands is indicated for evaluation of cystic, neoplastic, or other soft tissue changes in the parenchyma or surrounding glandular tissue (see chapter 1). MRI can also be used to perform sialographic studies, providing greater resolution and a three-dimensional image compared to standard sialography.

8.2.4.5 *Sialoendoscopy*

Sialoendoscopy is both a diagnostic and interventional technique that permits the direct visualization and removal of sialoliths when located in the proximal aspect of the excretory duct. A small fiber-optic endoscope is inserted through the major salivary gland duct orifice to identify the sialolith and remove it using a variety of methods (lithotripsy, laser fragmentation, basket removal). The main disadvantage of this procedure is its clinical limitations (cannot access beyond tertiary ducts) and the risk of duct perforation.

8.2.5 *Other diagnostic modalities*

Salivary gland biopsy may be warranted to rule-out neoplastic disease (see chapter 9) or as part of the tests to diagnose Sjögren syndrome. A major gland biopsy is an invasive procedure that usually requires an extraoral approach, and care must be taken by the surgeon to avoid severing the duct and adjacent structures. Fine needle aspiration (see chapter 9) is a less invasive alternative procedure that may be used preliminarily to evaluate major salivary gland tissues when there is concern for malignancy. This procedure involves obtaining a small sample of cells for cytopathologic evaluation; however, there is likelihood that sampling error may produce false negative results. A patient who requires biopsy of a major salivary gland should be referred to an oral or head and neck surgeon for further evaluation and management.

Minor salivary gland biopsy is a simple and relatively low-risk surgical procedure. It is the preferred choice of biopsy when considering a diagnosis of Sjögren syndrome. This procedure is performed by making a small incision in the lower labial mucosa and dissecting out six to eight minor salivary glands that are submitted for histopathologic evaluation.

8.3 Diagnosis of salivary gland disorders

8.3.1 *Sialolithiasis*

Sialolithiasis, or salivary stone formation, can lead to partial or complete obstruction of salivary flow and is often associated with secondary sialadenitis. A common clinical presentation is intermittent painful enlargement of the affected gland associated with food intake,

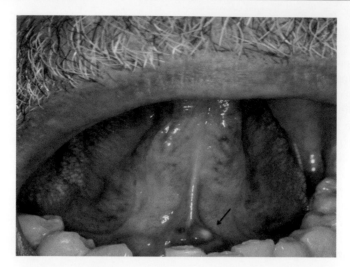

Figure 8.4   Sialolith causing salivary gland obstruction in a 63-year-old male complaining of acute pain in the left floor of the mouth. Note the positioning of the sialolith close to the duct orifice.

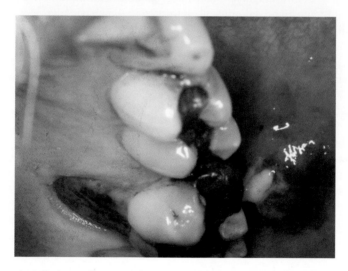

Figure 8.5   Purulent discharge from the left Stensen duct orifice in a 43-year-old male with a previous history of recurrent duct obstruction secondary to sialolithiasis.

with symptoms ranging from mild burning to sharp pain. Sialoliths can develop within minor and major salivary glands and are most frequently encountered in the submandibular ductal system (Figure 8.4). Stones can often be palpated when examining the anatomy of the salivary ducts. In some circumstances, calcifications may be directly visualized when they are located proximal to the duct orifice, in which they may appear as one or more yellow to white firm stone-like structures. In addition to pain and obstruction, retrograde secondary bacterial infection of the gland may occur (Figure 8.5). Radiographic evaluation should begin with an occlusal and/or panoramic image; however, computed tomography (CT) may be indicated in some circumstances (see chapter 1). The degree of calcification varies greatly, and consequently some stones will not be visible radiographically.

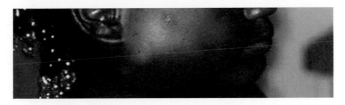

Figure 8.6 Acute parotid gland swelling in a 9-year-old female diagnosed with Sjögren syndrome, with an 18-month history of intermittent bilateral swelling and recurrent glandular infection.

8.3.2 Sialadenitis

Sialadenitis is defined as inflammation of the minor or major salivary glands and is characterized by mild to moderate pain that may or may not be related to food intake. This condition is seen in association with dehydration and radiation treatment, as well as autoimmune and granulomatous disease. In smokers, transient sialadenitis of the palatal minor salivary glands ("nicotine stomatitis" or "smoker's palate") may be evident, characterized by ductal dilation and papillary inflammatory mucosal changes. In patients with Sjögren syndrome, sialadenitis of the parotid glands is common and may present with bilateral gland swelling that is visible extraorally. The diagnosis of sialadenitis is based primarily on clinical findings.

8.3.3 Salivary gland infections

Bacterial infection of the major salivary glands typically involves a single gland and is characterized by extraoral swelling and erythema, intense pain, and the presence of purulent exudate (fluid that is not clear in color) from the duct orifice upon stimulation (Figure 8.5 and 8.6; see chapter 1). Systemic signs such as fever and chills may also be present. This acute suppurative infection warrants management with antibiotics. If the infection persists despite an adequate course of antibiotics, the exudate should be submitted for culture and susceptibility testing (see chapter 7). Debilitated patients and those with severe salivary gland hypofunction are at highest risk. Viral infections that may affect the salivary glands are discussed in chapter 7.

8.3.4 Mucocele

A mucocele, or *mucous extravasation phenomenon*, is a benign lesion caused by the damage and/or severance of one or more minor salivary gland ducts. These lesions appear on the mucosa as raised, fluid-filled dome-shaped masses that are translucent to blue in color depending on the depth of the lesion (Figure 8.7). These may become fibrotic over time if not removed. The most common location for a mucocele is the lower lip due to frequent bite injury, though the buccal mucosa, lateral tongue, and soft palate may be affected. A mucocele located on the floor of the mouth is called a *ranula*, caused by damage to the sublingual gland (Figure 8.8). The diagnosis of a mucocele is based on clinical findings; however, persistent lesions require surgical excision, and all specimens should be submitted for routine histopathology.

8.3.5 Necrotizing sialometaplasia

Necrotizing sialometaplasia is a rare condition that presents as an acute deep, necrotic-appearing ulceration of the hard palate with raised indurated borders (Figure 8.9). It is typically associated with a history of trauma to the area, such as a dental injection, chemical

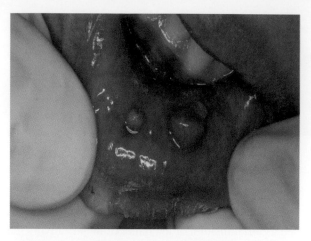

Figure 8.7 Two mucoceles on the lower lip of a 14-year-old female with a history of factitious lip biting.

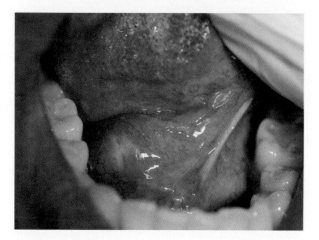

Figure 8.8 Ranula of the right sublingual gland in a 28-year-old male with a recent history of traumatic perforating injury to the floor of the mouth.

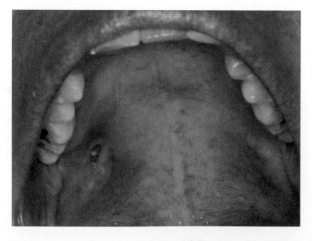

Figure 8.9 Necrotizing sialometaplasia that developed following administration of a local anesthetic block to the right palate of a 32-year-old female.

burn, injury while eating, or iatrogenic injury in patients with bulimia. Necrotizing sialometaplasia is a self-limiting condition that heals within 6–8 weeks. Its appearance and unilateral presentation often lead clinicians to suspect malignancy (see chapter 9), and if no clinical improvement is noted within 2 weeks, a biopsy should be obtained from the margin of the lesion, including affected and unaffected tissue. Histopathologic evaluation by an oral pathologist is recommended.

8.3.6 Sialadenosis

Sialadenosis is a non-inflammatory disorder characterized by salivary gland enlargement that most frequently affects the parotid glands. The clinical presentation is a persistent, asymptomatic, bilateral enlargement of the affected glands. This disorder is typically associated with one or multiple underlying systemic conditions, including diabetes mellitus or other endocrinopathies, malnutrition syndrome, or alcoholism. Sialadenosis may result secondary to sympathetic denervation of the salivary acini, leading to excessive intracellular accumulation of secretory granules and enlargement of the acinar cells; however, the etiology remains unknown. Definitive diagnosis may require imaging studies such as sialography, CT (see chapter 1), or salivary gland biopsy to differentiate it from an inflammatory or neoplastic condition.

8.3.7 Sarcoidosis

Sarcoidosis is a granulomatous disease in which collections of chronic inflammatory cells (granulomas) form as nodules in multiple organs. Sarcoidosis most commonly presents in the lungs or lymph nodes, but virtually any organ, including the salivary glands, can be affected. The diagnostic work-up for sarcoidosis is described in chapter 11.

8.4 Sjögren syndrome

Sjögren syndrome is an autoimmune disease characterized by systemic inflammation and decreased function of the salivary and lacrimal glands, resulting in oral and ocular dryness (Figure 8.10). The disorder is most prevalent in middle-aged females, with the female-to-male ratio being approximately 9:1. The combination of complaints of oral dryness and ocular symptoms (dryness, sandy feeling under the eyelids) is known as the *sicca complex* or *sicca syndrome*. The underlying pathophysiology of Sjögren syndrome involves dysregulated B-cell activity, development of autoantibodies against multiple self-antigens, and an intense T-cell infiltration of major exocrine glands. Oral sequelae include xerostomia and salivary hypofunction, oral burning, and an increased risk of candidiasis and rampant dental caries. Sjögren syndrome may occur in patients who have an already diagnosed concomitant autoimmune disease, with the most common being rheumatoid arthritis, systemic lupus erythematosus, and chronic autoimmune hepatitis.

8.4.1 Diagnostic criteria

Standardized European-American criteria for the diagnosis of Sjögren syndrome were published in 2002, based on clinical (oral/ocular symptoms and signs), serologic, and histopathologic criteria (Table 8.3). A diagnostic update published in 2012 by the Sjögren's International Collaborative Clinical Alliance (SICCA) was endorsed by the American College of Rheumatology and considers only objective measures to diagnose the disease.

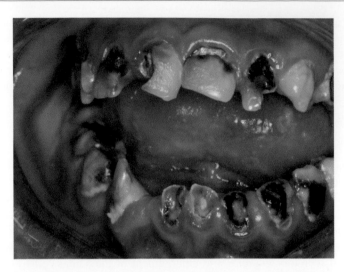

Figure 8.10 16-year-old female diagnosed with Sjögren syndrome, presenting with severe hyposalivation, erythematous soft tissues, and rampant dental caries.

Using this revised classification criteria, a diagnosis of Sjögren syndrome is established if at least two of three objective criteria are positive (Table 8.4).

8.4.1.1 *Oral signs and symptoms*

Patients with Sjögren syndrome may present with characteristic oral findings, such as severe salivary gland hypofunction and persistent bilateral sialadenitis. Oral signs that contribute to a diagnosis of Sjögren syndrome include an unstimulated whole salivary gland flow of 1.5 mL or less in 5 minutes (section 8.2.1), parotid sialography showing the presence of diffuse sialectasia (punctate, cavitary, or destructive pattern; section 8.2.4.1) without evidence of obstruction in the major duct(s), and/or salivary scintigraphy with delayed uptake, reduced concentration, or delayed excretion of tracer (section 8.2.4.3). In clinical practice however, these diagnostic measures are rarely ordered. Symptoms of Sjögren syndrome include complaints of xerostomia for at least 3 months and requiring liquids to swallow dry foods. Sialadenitis of the major salivary glands is common and may be associated with chronic pain.

8.4.1.2 *Ocular signs and symptoms*

Ocular tests for Sjögren syndrome assess objective evidence of ocular dryness. The *Schirmer test* uses absorbent paper strips that measure tear film production over a 5-minute period, with greater than 5 millimeters (mm) on the test strip being considered "normal," and anything less considered "abnormal" or "low." The *Rose Bengal test* assists the ophthalmologist in evaluating the cornea and conjunctiva for abrasions. This test relies on the application of a sodium salt-based resorbable dye that stains corneal and conjunctival damaged cells, and results are determined using a scoring system. An alternate test endorsed by the SICCA cohort utilizes fluorescein staining to grade the cornea and lissamine green staining to grade nasal and bulbar conjunctivae. The SICCA *ocular staining score* is a grading system used to quantify ocular surface staining. Symptoms of ocular dryness include a complaint of dry eyes for at least 3 months, a foreign body sensation in the eyes, and the use of artificial tears more than three times per day.

Table 8.3 European-American criteria for diagnosis of Sjögren syndrome.*,†

Ocular findings	Oral findings	Histopathologic findings	Serology
Signs (at least 1) – Schirmer test, (without anesthesia) ≤ 5 mm/5 min – Positive ocular dye staining (van Bijsterveld score ≥ 4) Symptoms (at least 1) – Dry eyes > 3 months – Foreign body sensation in the eyes – Use of artificial tears > 3× per day	Signs (at least 1) – Unstimulated whole salivary flow ≤ 1.5 mL/15 min – Parotid sialography with diffuse sialectasias and no obstruction in major ducts – Salivary scintigraphy with delayed uptake, reduced concentration and/or delayed excretion of tracer Symptoms (at least 1) – Dry mouth > 3 months – Recurrent or persistently swollen salivary glands – Need liquids to swallow dry foods	– Focal lymphocytic sialoadenitis with focus score ≥ 1	– >25 units/mL of antibodies to SSA (Ro), and/or – >25 units/mL of antibodies to SSB (La)

*For a diagnosis of primary Sjögren syndrome, any 4 of the 6 (ocular/oral signs, ocular/oral symptoms, histopathology or serology) criteria must be present, including either histopathology or serology, or any 3 of the 4 objective criteria (ocular/oral signs, histology, serology). For a Sjögren syndrome diagnosis in patients with another well-defined major connective tissue disease, the presence of 1 symptom (ocular/oral) plus 2 of the 3 objective criteria (ocular/oral signs, histology) is diagnostic.
†Reference: Vitali C, Bombardieri S, Jonsson R, et al. Classification criteria for Sjögren's syndrome: A revised version of the European criteria proposed by the American-European Consensus Group. Ann Rheum Dis 2002;61(6):554–558.

Table 8.4 Sjögren's International Collaborative Clinical Alliance (SICCA) classification criteria for Sjögren syndrome.*

Classification of SS will be met in patients who have at least 2 of the following 3 objective features:
Serology
– Positive serum anti-SSA/Ro and/or anti-SSB/La OR
– Positive rheumatoid factor AND ANA titer ≥ 1:320
Objective oral (histopathologic) criteria
– Labial salivary gland biopsy exhibiting focal lymphocytic sialadenitis with a focus score ≥ 1 focus/4 mm^2
Objective ocular criteria
– Keratoconjunctivitis sicca with ocular staining score ≥ 3[†]

*Shiboski SC, Shiboski CH, Criswell L, et al. Sjögren's International Collaborative Clinical Alliance (SICCA) Research Groups. American College of Rheumatology classification criteria for Sjögren's syndrome: A data-driven, expert consensus approach in the Sjögren's International Collaborative Clinical Alliance cohort. Arthritis Care Res 2012;64: 475–487.
[†]Assuming the individual is not currently using daily eye drops for glaucoma and has not had corneal surgery or cosmetic eyelid surgery in the last 5 years.

Table 8.5 Serology for salivary gland disorders.

Test	Normal values	Clinical significance
Antinuclear antibodies (ANA)	titer < 1:160	If titer ≥ 1:160, supportive of autoimmune disease
Angiotensin-converting enzyme (ACE) levels	8–53 units/L	> 53 units/L, supportive of glandular involvement secondary to sarcoidosis
Anti-SSA, Anti-SSB	< 20 units/mL	> 25 units/mL of either is one criterion for SS
Rheumatoid factor (RF)	< 30 units/mL	If > 30 U, supportive of autoimmune disease
Sedimentation rate (ESR)	Male: age/2 in mm/hr; female: (age +10)/2 in mm/hr	If > 30 mm/hr, non-specific inflammation, may be associated with autoimmune disease

8.4.1.3 *Serology*

Serology can be used to evaluate for evidence of autoimmune disease. The two autoantibodies that are the most highly associated with a diagnosis of Sjögren syndrome are anti-SSa, also known as anti-Ro, and anti-SSb, or anti-La, and positive values (greater than 25 units per mL) of one or both are serologic variables included in the diagnostic criteria for Sjögren syndrome. The SICCA classification criteria utilizes other markers as an alternative to fulfill the serologic criteria for Sjögren syndrome, specifically a positive rheumatoid factor and highly positive antinuclear antibody (ANA) test (Tables 8.4 and 8.5; see chapter 11).

8.4.1.4 *Minor salivary gland biopsy*

A salivary gland biopsy can provide histopathologic criteria to aid in the diagnosis of Sjögren syndrome (section 8.2.5). Characteristic findings include a multifocal dense, lymphocytic infiltration of the salivary gland tissue that may be present in both minor and major glands. The lymphocytic infiltrate surrounding the gland parenchyma is quantified as a *focus score*, defined as the number of lymphocytic foci (containing more than 50 lymphocytes) per $4\,mm^2$ of glandular tissue, adjacent to otherwise normal-appearing mucous acini. A focus score greater than or equal to one is a positive histopathologic finding for Sjögren syndrome and differentiates this condition from other causes of non-specific inflammation, where the lymphocytic infiltrate is more diffuse. Minor salivary gland biopsy specimens should be sent to an experienced oral pathologist for appropriate assessment of the focus score.

8.5 Suggested literature

Capaccio P, Cuccarini V, Ottaviani F, Minorati D, Sambataro G, Cornalba P, et al. Comparative ultrasonographic, magnetic resonance sialographic, and videoendoscopic assessment of salivary duct disorders. Ann Otol Rhinol Laryngol 2008;117:245–252.

Drage NA, Brown JE. Cone beam computed sialography of sialoliths. Dentomaxillofac Radiol 2009 Jul;38:301–305.

Navazesh M, Kumar SK. Measuring salivary flow: Challenges and opportunities. JADA 2008 May;139 Suppl:35 S–40 S.

Navazesh M, Christensen C, Brightman V. Clinical criteria for the diagnosis of salivary gland hypofunction. J Dent Res 1992 Jul;71:1363–1369.

Shiboski SC, Shiboski CH, Criswell L, et al. Sjögren's International Collaborative Clinical Alliance (SICCA) Research Groups. American College of Rheumatology classification criteria for Sjögren's syndrome: A data-driven, expert consensus approach in the Sjögren's International Collaborative Clinical Alliance Cohort. Arthritis Care Res 2012;64:475–487.

Thomson WM, Chalmers JM, Spencer AJ, Slade GD. Medication and dry mouth: Findings from a cohort study of older people. J Public Health Dent 2000 Winter;60:12–20.

Thomson WM, Chalmers JM, Spencer AJ, Williams SM. The Xerostomia Inventory: A multi-item approach to measuring dry mouth. Community Dent Health 1999;16:12–17.

Turner MD, Ship JA. Dry mouth and its effects on the oral health of elderly people. JADA 2007 Sep;138 Suppl:15 S–20 S.

Vinagre F, Santos MJ, Prata A, da Silva JC, Santos AI. Assessment of salivary gland function in Sjögren's syndrome: The role of salivary gland scintigraphy. Autoimmun Rev 2009;8:672–676.

Vitali C, Bombardieri S, Jonsson R, et al. Classification criteria for Sjögren's syndrome: A revised version of the European criteria proposed by the American-European Consensus Group. Ann Rheum Dis 2002;61(6):554–558.

9 Oral Neoplastic Disease

9.0 INTRODUCTION

Both benign and malignant neoplastic conditions can be encountered in the oral cavity, potentially making oral health care specialists primarily responsible for initial detection of such lesions. Similarly, oral health care providers play an important role in surveillance of patients who have previously been treated for head and neck cancer given the high risk of local recurrence and new primary tumors. Importantly, earlier diagnosis of neoplastic disease can have a significant impact on improving treatment outcomes and therefore reducing a patient's morbidity and mortality. Tumors can arise from any tissue component of the oral cavity, including squamous mucosa, salivary glands, bone and cartilage, teeth, muscle, fibrous tissue, vascular tissue, neural tissue, and fat (Table 9.1). In addition to primary diseases arising within the oral cavity, metastatic tumors and hematologic malignancies can present with oral signs and symptoms, and these findings may represent the initial clinical manifestation or may indicate recurrent/relapsed disease.

Oral neoplastic disease can present with a range of signs and symptoms that generally correspond to the size, location, and extent of disease, as well as specific clinical features that are unique to certain conditions (Alert Box 9.1). Pain is generally caused by nerve involvement and may be encountered at any stage of disease. Jaw asymmetry, limited mouth opening (trismus), shifting and/or loosening of teeth, a change in the fit of a removable prosthesis, and paresthesia or other neurosensory changes can all be signs of benign or malignant tumors. When present, symptoms may be constant or episodic and may be provoked by functional movements such as speaking, chewing, or swallowing. Paresthesia or anesthesia is generally an ominous sign suggestive of invasive disease, and neurosensory changes in the cranial and/or cervical nerve distribution should be considered highly suspicious for a primary tumor or metastasis to the head and/or neck. Of particular note, metastasis to the mandible should be considered if neurosensory changes present in the mental nerve distribution, especially in a patient with a known history of a solid cancer (e.g., breast, lung, prostate), with or without a known history of metastases (Figure 9.1). Loss of motor function, manifested by difficulty speaking, chewing, or swallowing, is another important potential sign of malignancy that can be observed in the context of both local/intraoral (e.g., squamous cell carcinoma of the tongue) and central (e.g., metastatic disease to the brain; Figure 9.2) lesions. Soft tissue

Risk Assessment and Oral Diagnostics in Clinical Dentistry, First Edition.
Dena J. Fischer, Nathaniel S. Treister and Andres Pinto.
© 2013 John Wiley & Sons, Inc. Published 2013 by John Wiley & Sons, Inc.

Table 9.1 Benign and malignant tumors of the head and neck.

	Tumor	Cell/Tissue of origin	Special features
Benign Neoplasms	Ameloblastoma	Odontogenic epithelium	Most common odontogenic neoplasm; multilocular radiolucencies; some subtypes may demonstrate malignant features histopathologically
	Cementoblastoma	Cementoblasts	Rare; pain and swelling common; periradicular radiopacity
	Granular cell tumor	Unknown	Tongue most common site in body; asymptomatic subepithelial nodule
	Lipoma	Adipose tissue	Soft, smooth, painless nodule
	Myxoma	Odontogenic ectomesenchyme	Unilocular or multilocular radiolucency
	Neurofibroma	Schwann cells and perineural fibroblasts	Slow-growing, soft, painless mass; can develop in bone
	Ossifying fibroma	Bone tissue	Painless, enlarging unilocular radiolucency
	Osteoblastoma	Osteoblasts	Rare; pain and swelling common; radiolucent with mineralization evident
	Pleomorphic adenoma	Salivary gland	Painless and slow growing; long-term risk of malignant transformation (*carcinoma ex pleomorphic adenoma*)
	Rhabdomyoma	Skeletal muscle	Rare
	Schwannoma	Schwann cells	Slow growing; arises from nerve trunk; generally asymptomatic
Malignant Neoplasms	Adenoid cystic carcinoma	Salivary gland	Pain common due to perineural invasion
	Angiosarcoma	Endothelium	Oral lesions rare, but 50% occur in head and neck region
	Chondrosarcoma	Cartilage	Rare, can effect TMJ
	Kaposi sarcoma	Endothelium	HHV8; associated with HIV/AIDS
	Melanoma	Melanocytes	Generally pigmented; unrelated to sun exposure in oral cavity; very rare and very poor prognosis
	Mucoepidermoid carcinoma	Salivary gland	Most common salivary gland malignancy
	Osteosarcoma	Bone	"Sunburst" pattern of bone trabeculation
	Rhabdomyosarcoma	Skeletal muscle	Most common soft tissue sarcoma in children; 40% involve head and neck
	Squamous cell carcinoma	Squamous epithelium	Most common oral malignancy; wide range of clinical features
	Verrucous carcinoma	Squamous epithelium	Thick white papillary plaque; often develops in area of leukoplakia

changes that should be considered suspicious include focal areas of thickening and/or mass-like changes, non-healing ulcerations, and induration. Periapical and panoramic radiographic features of neoplastic disease include focal areas of radiolucency and radiopacity, focal destruction of cortical bone, and the appearance of "floating" teeth (Figure 9.3).

Alert Box 9.1   Signs/symptoms suggestive of oral malignant disease.

Clinical signs	Clinical symptoms
White and red changes (erythroleukoplakia)	Pain
Ulceration	Paresthesia/sensory changes
Induration	Bleeding
Exophytic/endophytic growth	Motor changes
Change in fit of oral prosthesis	Dysphagia
Unexplained mobility of teeth	
Neurologic abnormalities	

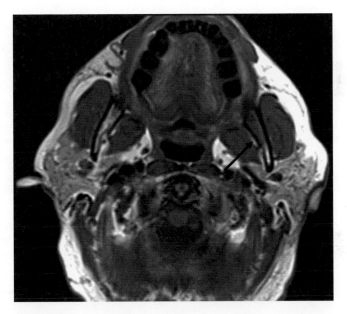

Figure 9.1   57-year-old male with diffuse large B-cell lymphoma with acute onset of pain and paresthesia of the left posterior mandible and ramus. Axial T1-weighted MRI of the brain demonstrated unusual appearance of the marrow in the left mandible near the area of the inferior alveolar nerve foramen, with prolonged T1 and T2 signal, consistent with marrow infiltration of his underlying lymphoma.

Nearly 95% of all oral malignancies are squamous cell carcinomas (SCCs) that arise from the mucosal lining of the oral cavity. Lymphoma, salivary gland cancers, and other less common malignancies, as well as distant metastases to the oral cavity, account for the remainder. Relative to many of the other conditions discussed in this book, cancer is a very rare disease; however, the consequences of a delay in diagnosis or misdiagnosis can be devastating. Therefore, it is imperative for oral health care specialists to recognize signs and symptoms and to provide appropriate and timely referral for diagnosis and comprehensive management.

More challenging is the diagnosis and management of *pre-malignant* or what are often more appropriately termed *potentially malignant* oral lesions, defined as lesions that have the potential to undergo malignant transformation. The goal of the oral health care provider should be to facilitate diagnosis and to reduce as much as possible any lag time between

(a)

(b)

(c)

(d)

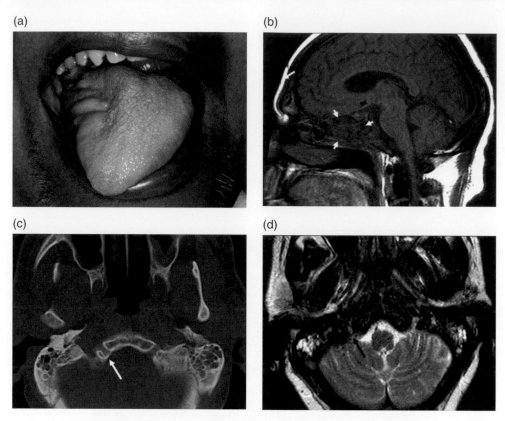

Figure 9.2   62-year-old male with metastatic prostate cancer with progressive right-sided tongue and constrictor muscle weakness (patient is moving the tongue as far to the right as possible) and difficulty speaking and swallowing (a). Sagittal MRI (b) demonstrates the extent of the metastatic lesion in the area of the clivus. Axial images demonstrate narrowing of the outlet of the right cranial nerve XII (computed tomography; c), and cranial nerve IX (MRI; d).

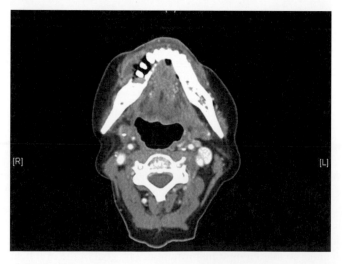

Figure 9.3   Axial CT scan of a patient with advanced relapsed squamous cell carcinoma of the right mandible with destruction of the cortical bone.

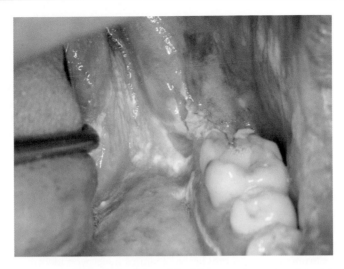

Figure 9.4   Proliferative verrucous leukoplakia of the left retromolar pad, mylohyoid ridge, and lateral tongue.

detection of clinical abnormalities and referral to a specialist for close monitoring, diagnosis, and/or further management.

9.1   Benign neoplasms of the oral cavity

Benign neoplasms can arise from any tissue type and have unlimited growth potential. Despite being "benign," such lesions may be associated with significant morbidity, depending on the size and location of the lesion and the approach for management. Many neoplasms will present asymptomatically, being detected during routine clinical or radiographic examination. Regardless of clinical features, all suspicious lesions require biopsy for definitive diagnosis, and further testing may be warranted to determine the most appropriate management.

9.2   Oral potentially malignant lesions

Oral potentially malignant lesions include *leukoplakia, erythroleukoplakia*, and *erythroplakia*. Leukoplakia is defined as a white mucosal plaque that cannot be removed and cannot be diagnosed as any other condition (e.g., lichen planus, pseudomembranous candidiasis). The risk that leukoplakia will undergo malignant transformation over a patient's lifetime ranges from less than 5% to as high as 40%; however, no reliable indicators have been identified that can actually predict this risk. *Proliferative verrucous leukoplakia* is a unique clinical entity seen primarily in older women, characterized by one or more areas of folded/wrinkled-appearing leukoplakia (Figure 9.4) that extend slowly with time; it is associated with a high rate of malignant transformation to verrucous carcinoma (a low-grade variant of SCC with low risk of metastasis) or SCC. *Erythroplakia* is defined as a red oral mucosal plaque that, like leukoplakia, cannot be defined as any other clinical entity (e.g., lichen planus, erythematous candidiasis). Erythroplakia and erythroleukoplakia (mixed red and white lesion) are associated with a very high risk of malignancy (much higher than leukoplakia), with as many as 90–100% of cases ultimately demonstrating severe dysplasia (carcinoma in situ) or transformation to invasive carcinoma.

The actual histopathologic diagnosis of any given potentially malignant lesion must also be considered to determine an overall assessment of cancer risk; therefore, biopsy of any suspicious lesion is essential. Microscopic findings can include normal-appearing epithelium, acanthosis (an orderly increase in thickness of the epithelium), hyperkeratosis, hyperplasia, dysplasia (disorderly cellular architecture with malignant features, including mitotic figures and pleomorphism), and SCC (same cellular changes as dysplasia with evidence of invasion through the basement membrane into the connective tissue). Dysplasia is typically graded based on the percentage of the epithelium affected as mild (1/3), moderate (2/3), or severe (synonymous with carcinoma in situ; full-thickness dysplasia but without invasion). Unfortunately, studies have demonstrated poor consistency in grading among pathologists. An inflammatory infiltrate at the junction of the basement membrane and underlying connective tissue can be seen variably, although the significance is unclear. To complicate matters further, chronic inflammation (i.e., in the context of oral lichen planus) can lead to secondary reactive cellular atypia that is frequently interpreted as "mild dysplasia." A number of genetic (e.g., p53 mutations), cytogenetic (e.g., loss of heterozygosity), and epigenetic (e.g., chromatin hypermethylation) features have been identified throughout the spectrum of histopathologic findings; however, none of these have proven to be reliable markers to indicate a greater or lesser risk of malignant transformation, although this continues to be an area of active research.

There is no consensus as to the optimal approach for management of oral potentially malignant lesions. Close surveillance with routine exams (at least every 6 months) is essential.

9.3 Oral squamous cell carcinoma

Squamous cell carcinoma of the oral cavity can be a potentially devastating disease associated with significant morbidity and mortality, especially when the cancer is diagnosed at an advanced stage. Aside from some very rare genetic disorders that predispose patients to developing oral squamous cell carcinoma, such as *dyskeratosis congenita* and *Fanconi anemia* (see chapter 2), the main risk factors are heavy smoking and alcohol consumption. A role for HPV infection has also been recently identified and is discussed below. There is a wide range of clinical presentations, with lesions appearing flat/raised, exophytic/endophytic, ulcerated/non-ulcerated, normal to red/white in color, and with/without associated pain or other symptoms (Figure 9.5). The 5-year survival rate for early stage localized oral cancer is over 80%; however, this figure falls to approximately 50% once there is regional lymph node involvement, and decreases further to only 30% when distant metastasis is detected. Depending on the location, extent, and stage of disease, treatment involves surgery and/or combined chemotherapy/radiation therapy. Complications of treatment include severe salivary gland hypofunction, trismus, chronic pain, and an increased risk of dental caries (see chapters 8 and 10). Importantly, patients with a history of oral SCC are at significantly elevated risk for localized recurrence as well as new primary lesions; therefore, vigilant long-term follow-up with an oncologist is mandatory.

High-risk HPV strains, particularly HPV16 (identified histopathologically by immunohistochemical and in situ hybridization techniques), are associated with cancers of the oropharynx, particularly the tonsils and base of the tongue. The clinical epidemiology is also unique in that these cancers may be encountered in younger patients, often without a history of tobacco or alcohol abuse. These oropharyngeal cancers are usually occult within lymphoepithelial tissue and therefore tend to be diagnosed at late stages, often with metastatic disease in the neck lymph nodes as the initial presentation. Importantly, these cancers

(a)   (b)

(c)   (d)

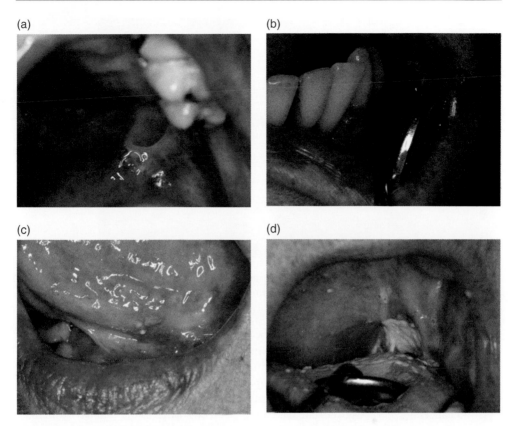

Figure 9.5 Squamous cell carcinomas of the oral cavity. (a) Ulceration and extensive erythematous changes of the left maxilla secondary to SCC arising from the maxillary sinus; (b) multifocal SCC of the facial gingiva and anterior buccal mucosa with an exophytic growth pattern; (c) recurrent SCC of the left ventrolateral tongue with a slightly exophytic ulcerative component and white changes; (d) ulcerative SCC of the left tonsil.

appear to be more radiosensitive, with significantly higher 5-year survival rates compared to HPV-negative cancers. The natural history of oral and oropharyngeal infection and persistence of HPV infection is poorly characterized, and the potential benefit of the HPV vaccine in preventing oropharyngeal SCC at this point remains speculative. Of note, benign HPV-associated oral lesions (e.g., squamous papilloma, verruca vulgaris) are not associated with a risk of malignant transformation. Based on these findings, oncologists now routinely evaluate SCC tissue for HPV positivity, and research is ongoing to study outcomes of modified treatment regimens based on HPV tumor status.

9.4   Other cancers of the oral cavity

Although occurring far less frequently than SCC, a variety of other malignancies arising from local tissues or metastatic from distant sites may be encountered in the oral cavity (Table 9.1). Salivary gland cancers can develop in the major or minor salivary glands and can present with swelling, erythema, and/or ulceration in the location of minor/major salivary glands, with variable symptoms including pain, paresthesia, and anesthesia.

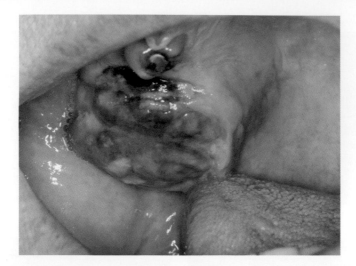

Figure 9.6 Extranodal presentation of non-Hodgkin lymphoma with a large mass-like ulceration of the posterior right maxilla and associated tooth mobility and pain.

Melanoma is rare in the oral cavity but must be considered when a new area of pigmentation is detected, especially when the borders are irregular and there are notable changes in the size and appearance over a short period of time. Other soft tissue carcinomas include sarcomas arising from various soft tissue components (e.g., muscle, vasculature); they are extremely rare and may present similarly to salivary gland cancers.

Solid cancers (e.g., breast, prostate, and lung) can metastasize to the oral cavity, in most cases to the bone of the mandible and gingiva, with other areas of soft tissue involvement being far less common. In addition, solid cancers may cause secondary oral signs/symptoms when there is neural involvement, for example, when the vagus or cranial nerves are affected (Figure 9.2). Hematologic malignancies may also initially present in the oral cavity, or the oral cavity may be a site of disease relapse. Lymphoma may present with neck lymphadenopathy or unilateral enlargement of the tonsils, or extranodally as a localized tissue swelling and/or ulceration within the oral cavity, usually the palate or the gingiva (Figure 9.6). Leukemia may present with prominent generalized gingival involvement characterized by erythematous and often painful overgrowth and/or swelling (Figure 9.7). In all cases, the clinical signs and symptoms, along with information obtained from the medical history, should guide further radiographic and/or histopathologic evaluation.

9.5 Diagnostic tests

9.5.1 Physical examination

Extraoral examination may detect growths and asymmetry, but this is not typically noted until tumors have grown to be very large. In addition, careful palpation of the submental, submandibular, and cervical lymph nodes may identify enlarged, firm, fixed lymphadenopathy that should be considered highly suspicious for regional lymph node metastasis. Nearly all epithelial abnormalities (including malignancy) in the oral cavity can be detected by careful visual inspection using a good light source and manual palpation; however, when symptoms or clinical concerns involve the oropharynx, referral to an otolaryngologist is

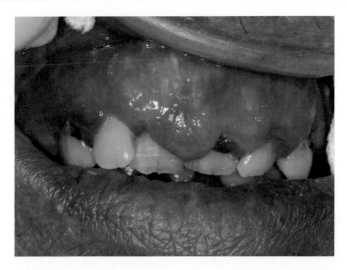

Figure 9.7 Gingival involvement in a patient with acute myelogenous leukemia, with sheet-like overgrowth and focal areas of hemorrhage.

(a)   (b)

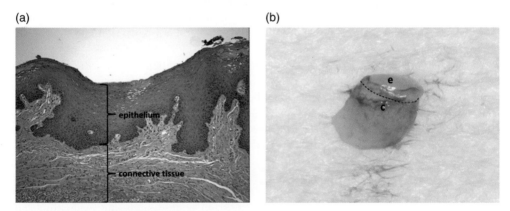

Figure 9.8 Punch biopsy of the oral mucosa including normal histopathology (a) and the surgical specimen (b), demonstrating full thickness of epithelium (e) and connective tissue (c) Sufficient depth of the biopsy is necessary to assess for evidence of invasion beyond the basement membrane.

warranted. Persistent white, red, mixed white/red, pigmented, and/or ulcerative lesions that are exophytic, flat, or endophytic, with or without induration (firmness), and that cannot obviously be attributed to a different diagnosis (e.g., cheek biting, lichen planus, geographic tongue) require biopsy. There is no substitute for a comprehensive extraoral and intraoral examination at routine intervals (i.e., dental recall appointments), as this is considered the gold standard screening test for detection of oral cancer.

9.5.2   Tissue biopsy

Tissue biopsy with histopathologic evaluation by a pathologist is the gold standard for diagnosis of cancer. The pathologist is limited by the quality and extent of the submitted tissue sample; therefore, it is critical that a full-thickness (i.e., includes epithelium and underlying connective tissue; Figure 9.8) representative sample is obtained by the clinician. In the case of large lesions, and especially those with multiple features (e.g., white, red, and ulcerated sections), multiple biopsies should be obtained, as invasive cancer may only be present focally, and the correct diagnosis can be missed due to sampling error. In most cases, the biopsy should be obtained from areas with "high-risk" features, including ulceration, induration, erythroleukoplakia, and verrucous or nodular morphology; depending on the size and location of the lesion, it may be beneficial to obtain a margin of clinically normal-appearing tissue to evaluate changes at the margins. Since the purpose of the biopsy is simply to obtain a diagnosis, but not to remove the lesion, a 4.0-millimeter punch biopsy is generally the easiest and most effective surgical instrument to use (see chapter 1). When there is any suspicion for malignancy, even in the case of small lesions (less than 0.5 centimeter), it is important to perform an incisional biopsy first to determine the diagnosis.

9.5.3   Cytology

Cytology plays a limited role in the diagnosis of malignancies of the oral cavity. Fine needle aspiration can be a useful diagnostic test to evaluate tissue that is not easily accessible, for example, an intrabony lesion, an enlarged parotid gland, or a swollen lymph node. This procedure is typically performed by a cytopathologist, sometimes with ultrasonography, to guide the needle biopsy to the correct site. The sample collected is simply a collection of cells without the structural context of a full-thickness biopsy, and findings must be carefully interpreted. This diagnostic technique requires expertise in both collection and interpretation of the cytology specimen.

Exfoliative full-thickness cytology (that includes basal epithelial cells) is not routinely used for the diagnosis of oral mucosal conditions and can never serve as a substitute for tissue biopsy. However, this technique may be of some benefit in patients who are being followed closely; for example, after treatment for oral cancer, when there are persistent clinical mucosal abnormalities that otherwise would not warrant frequent serial biopsies (e.g., every 1–3 months). This is an area of active research and is addressed in section 9.6.4.

9.5.4   Imaging studies

Imaging studies (see chapter 1) are routinely utilized in the diagnostic evaluation and work-up of oral tumors, in particular for staging malignancies and surveillance for recurrence and/or metastases. Computed tomography can be useful for determining the extent of tumor involvement, presence of bone invasion, proximity to vital structures, and lymph node involvement. Magnetic resonance imaging is the imaging modality of choice for soft tissue disease and is best used for assessment of salivary gland and other deep soft tissue tumors. When neurologic signs are suggestive of a central lesion, patients should be referred for a brain MRI (Figure 9.2). Positron emission tomography scanning, and in particular combined PET/CT imaging, is used routinely in oncology to identify areas of tumor activity, in particular for follow-up and restaging after treatment.

9.6   Adjunctive tests

In recent years, a range of adjunctive aids have been introduced and marketed to the dental community for the purpose of assisting in the early detection of potentially pre-malignant and malignant lesions. None of these adjunctive aids have been subjected to proper clinical evaluation to determine their true ability to detect such mucosal changes (as measured by sensitivity and specificity), in particular with respect to comparison with standard clinical examination and/or tissue biopsy. Importantly, the interpretation of non-neoplastic inflammatory oral pathologic conditions that are often associated with reactive epithelial atypia (e.g., oral lichen planus) has not been adequately evaluated with these adjunctive tests. There is no available data to suggest that these adjunctive aids should be used for indiscriminate screening of the general population, but they may play a limited role in helping to determine whether or not a lesion should be referred to a specialist for further evaluation or possibly to help guide biopsy site selection.

9.6.1   Chemoluminescence and tissue reflectance

Several devices have been designed based on the concept that mucosa undergoing abnormal malignant change reflects light differently than normal tissue. In the United States, these include Microlux/DL (AdDent, Danbury, CT), Orascoptic DK (Orascoptic, Middleton, WI), and ViziLite Plus (Zila Pharmaceuticals, Phoenix, AZ). With each system, the patient first rinses with a 1% acetic acid solution to permit better light transmission, and a blue-white light is then applied with visual inspection to look for what are termed "acetowhite" areas that can then be subjected to biopsy. The ViziLite Plus system also includes a toluidine blue solution (see section 9.6.3). *Recommendation: Tissue reflectance devices do not have a proven benefit over visual inspection with a good light source for the detection of potentially malignant and malignant oral lesions.*

9.6.2   Autofluorescence

VELscope (LED Dental, Burnaby, British Columbia, Canada) and Identifi 3000 (StarDental, Lancaster, PA) are FDA-approved devices that use autofluorescence technology. Normal tissue "autofluoresces" due to the presence of naturally occurring cellular "fluorophores" under intensive blue light (400–460 nm) excitation and appears pale green under provided glasses with a specific filter. Abnormal mucosa has decreased levels of autofluorescence and appears darker, thereby potentially identifying areas that should be subjected to biopsy. However, loss of autofluorescence is not limited to dysplasia/malignancy and can be seen in areas of inflammation as well. There is currently active research evaluating the utility of and potential clinical indications for VELscope as an adjunctive aid in the diagnosis of oral cancer. *Recommendation: Tissue autofluorescence devices do not have a proven benefit over visual inspection with a good light source for the detection of potentially malignant and malignant oral lesions. Tissue autofluorescence devices may be of some utility as an adjunctive aid in guiding biopsy site selection.*

9.6.3   Toluidine blue/tolonium chloride

Toluidine blue has been evaluated extensively for its ability to preferentially stain abnormal tissues and has been used as both a screening tool as well as an adjunctive aid for biopsy site selection. Toluidine blue stains cellular DNA in the superficial three to four layers of cells, so that cells with increased mitoses/genetic material appear as blue or purple. Research findings have overall been mixed, in part due to variable application techniques (brush on vs. rinse, various concentrations, etc.) and criteria for determining "positive" staining. It is important to note that cells that are in the process of active regeneration from inflammation (e.g., a bite injury) may demonstrate a similar staining pattern. *Recommendation: Toluidine blue does not have a proven benefit over visual inspection with a good light source for the detection of potentially malignant and malignant oral lesions. Toluidine blue may be of some utility as an adjunctive aid in guiding biopsy site selection.*

9.6.4 Oral brush cytology

The Oral CDx Brush Test (Oral CDx Laboratories, Suffren, NY) is a case-finding device for the detection of oral pre-malignant and malignant lesions. It is intended to be used primarily in cases where there is a low index of suspicion and tissue biopsy would not be performed. The provided kit includes a cytology brush that, when used appropriately, obtains a full-thickness sample of cells that are submitted for cytopathologic analysis. The specimen is interpreted as "normal," "atypical," or "positive," but a tissue diagnosis is not provided. Furthermore, atypical-appearing cells are commonly seen in the context of inflammation. *Recommendation: Any oral mucosal lesions that are suspicious for malignancy should be subjected to tissue biopsy.*

9.6.5 Summary of recommendations for the use of adjunctive tests

While there is cautious optimism among specialists, additional research is warranted before more definitive guidelines on the utility of adjunctive tests can be recommended. At this time, none of these tests appear to play a role in overall oral cancer screening, but specific tests may be of some benefit in certain clinical circumstances.

9.7 Selected literature

Gillison J, et al. Distinct risk factor profiles for human papillomavirus type 16-positive and human papillomavirus type 16-negative head and neck cancers. J Natl Cancer Inst 2008;100:407–420.

Karabulut A, et al. Observer variability in the histologic assessment of oral premalignant lesions. J Oral Pathol Med 1995;24:198–200.

Lingen M, et al. Critical evaluation of diagnostic aids for the detection of oral cancer. Oral Oncology 2008;44:10–22.

Pfister D, et al. Head and neck cancers: Clinical practice guidelines. J Natl Comp Cancer Network 2011;9:596–650.

Rethman M, et al. Evidence-based clinical recommendations regarding screening for oral squamous cell carcinomas. JADA 2010;141(5):509–520.

Shafer WG, Waldron CA. Erythroplakia of the oral cavity. Cancer 1975;36:1021–1028.

Van der Waal I. Potentially malignant disorders of the oral and oropharyngeal mucosa; terminology, classification and present concepts of management. Oral Oncology 2009;45:317–323.

Warnakulasuriya S, Johnson N, van der Waal I. Nomenclature and classification of potentially malignant disorders of the oral mucosa. J Oral Pathol Med 2007;36:575–580.

10 Oral Complications Associated with Cancer Therapy

10.0 INTRODUCTION

Treatment for cancer may result in short- and long-term changes that can adversely affect oral health, general health, and quality of life. Malignancies with the greatest potential to impact the oral cavity include head and neck cancers, hematologic cancers, and cancers that have metastasized to bone; however, almost any cancer, depending on the location and treatment, can potentially cause adverse oral effects. Oral complications may develop from direct damage to oral tissues as a result of surgery and/or radiation therapy (RT), as well as indirect damage due to regional or systemic toxicity associated with cytoreductive chemotherapy (CT), immunotherapy, and/or targeted molecular therapies. Even supportive care in cancer therapy can cause oral complications, such as hyposalivation due to use of opioid analgesics and medication-associated osteonecrosis of the jaw. Oral infections are common when salivary gland and/or immune function are compromised by cancer therapy and can exacerbate therapy-related toxicity to oral structures. With recent advances in the understanding of the basic biology of cancer and the increasing use of targeted molecular therapies, new oral complications are emerging that were not previously encountered in oncology; for example, aphthous-like stomatitis secondary to mammalian target of rapamycin (mTOR) inhibitors.

Oral complications can be characterized as acute or chronic (Table 10.1). Acute or early effects occur during the course of therapy and are primarily due to direct tissue toxicity. Acute reactions are generally self-limiting and typically resolve over weeks to months following the completion of therapy. Oral mucositis is a serious acute complication in which lesions of the oropharynx often precede the oral cavity. Mucositis may cluster with full-spectrum gastrointestinal toxicities to include nausea, vomiting, and diarrhea. Chronic or late effects occur months to years after completion of therapy, often when patients are in long-term remission from their primary cancer, and result in permanent tissue damage and lifelong morbidity that have a profound impact on overall health and quality of life. Oral health care providers play a key role in the prevention, identification, and management of such complications in cancer patients.

Risk Assessment and Oral Diagnostics in Clinical Dentistry, First Edition.
Dena J. Fischer, Nathaniel S. Treister and Andres Pinto.
© 2013 John Wiley & Sons, Inc. Published 2013 by John Wiley & Sons, Inc.

Table 10.1 Early and late effects of cancer treatment.

	Early effects	Early/late effects	Late effects
Radiotherapy	Oral mucositis Infection (bacterial, fungal, viral)	Hyposalivation Dysgeusia Dysosomnia Neuropathic pain	Neuropathic pain Caries PRON Fibrosis, trismus Dentofacial abnormalities[a] Recurrence, second primary, metastases
Chemotherapy	Oral mucositis Infection (bacterial, fungal, viral)	CIPN	CIPN ONJ[b] Dentofacial abnormalities[a] Recurrence, second primary, metastases
HSCT	Oral mucositis High risk for infection (bacterial, fungal, viral) Acute GVHD	Infections Chronic GVHD	Infections Chronic GVHD Caries Dentofacial abnormalities[a] ONJ[b, c] Relapse of underlying hematologic malignancy; PTLD Oral SCC

CIPN = chemotherapy-induced peripheral neuropathy.
GVHD = graft-versus-host disease.
HSCT = hematopoietic stem cell transplantation.
ONJ = medication-associated osteonecrosis of the jaws.
PRON = post-radiation osteonecrosis.
PTLD = post-transplant lymphoproliferative disorders.
SCC = squamous cell carcinoma.
[a] Limited to children only.
[b] If current or past history of antiresorptive medications.
[c] Patients on long-term steroid medications are often treated with antiresorptive medications for prevention of osteoporosis.

10.1 Cancer pre-treatment risk assessment

Prior to initiation of cancer therapy, the oral cavity should be carefully assessed and appropriate interventions should be provided to reduce the severity of oral complications during and after cancer treatment (Table 10.2). First, it is important to establish a rapport with the patient's oncology team and to have an understanding of the planned cancer treatment and potential complications. The most common cancers in the United States are solid tumors,

Table 10.2 Risk assessment prior to cancer treatment.

Complication	Procedures	Clinical Implications
Infection/bleeding following dental procedures	Evaluate laboratory values Consult with oncologist prior to performing dental treatment	Identify need for platelet transfusion or localized hemostatic measures Determine need for antibiotics Modification of treatment plan or timing of care
Infection during cancer treatment	Extraction of hopeless/non-restorable teeth Endodontic therapy/caries control Periodontal treatment	Eliminate/stabilize oral disease Anticipated periods of neutropenia
Mucosal injury	Smooth sharp edges of teeth and restorations Adjust ill-fitting prostheses	Impaired healing of soft tissues Increased risk of oral mucositis
Increased caries risk	Fabrication of fluoride trays and prescription-strength fluoride Oral hygiene instruction	Potential for salivary hypofunction Increased caries risk

Table 10.3 Potential causes of acute infection during cancer treatment.

- Dental caries extending to or approximating the pulp
- Active periodontal disease
- Symptomatic tooth
- Retained root
- Periapical pathology
- Recurrent episodes of pericoronitis

such as breast, lung, prostate, and/or colon cancers; these patients are generally considered to be at low risk for developing significant oral complications and are not typically evaluated prior to initiation of cancer treatment. Regardless, if CT is planned, individuals are at risk for the systemic toxic effects of various regimens. For these patients, potential causes of acute infections (Table 10.3) should be eliminated prior to treatment and patients should be evaluated during treatment if oral complications arise.

Individuals at a higher risk of developing early and/or late oral complications of cancer treatment include the following: (a) patients with head and neck cancers, including squamous cell carcinoma, salivary gland tumors, and extranodal (intraoral) lymphoma, (b) patients with hematologic malignancies, including leukemia, lymphoma, and multiple myeloma, and (c) patients treated with high-potency antiresorptive medications due to metastatic disease to the bone. In all of these high-risk patients, a comprehensive oral evaluation focused on minimizing the risk of oral complications should be completed. Necessary dental treatment should be delivered expeditiously, while providing adequate healing time for any surgical procedure, so that initiation of cancer treatment is not delayed. During the pre-treatment phase, the goal is to prevent acute infections or exacerbation of existing chronic oral infections during cancer treatment and to minimize the risk of complications arising during and post-therapy when patients may have complicated courses or remain immunosuppressed for extended periods.

10.1.1 *Head and neck cancers*

Patients undergoing treatment for head and neck cancer are typically treated with single modality therapy (e.g., surgery) or a combination of surgery, RT, and/or CT, all of which often contribute to the development of significant short- and long-term oral complications. Standard RT provides between 50 and 70 Gy (Gray unit—absorbed dose of radiation) cumulative dose, delivered in daily doses (fractionations) over 4–8 weeks. Patients who undergo RT to the head and neck have risks of long-term reduced healing capacity, tissue fibrosis, and salivary hypofunction due to permanent tissue damage. To improve tumor control and the risk of long-term treatment effects, advanced radiotherapy modalities and treatment regimens are being used for certain head and neck cancers. Intensity-modulated radiation therapy (IMRT) utilizes a three-dimensional dose distribution that spares normal tissues and reduces the volume of tissue exposed to radiation, thus reducing the risk for tissue toxicity. Other advanced treatment regimens for specific head and neck cancers (such as salivary gland) offer smaller and/or more frequent doses over a shorter period of time and have the capacity to improve tumor control while increasing the risk and severity of early and late RT effects. *Hyperfractionation*, the use of multiple smaller dose fractions, makes it possible to increase the total dose and increase the probability of tumor control. *Accelerated fractionation* typically involves twice daily dosing, which shortens the overall treatment time and minimizes the risk of tumor repopulation during treatment.

CT regimens are often administered concurrently with RT (*combined modality chemotherapy*) and have systemic toxic effects that may result in periods of immunosuppression. In some circumstances, *neoadjuvant* CT may be utilized initially to shrink the primary tumor prior to delivering other treatment, such as surgery or RT.

The pre-treatment phase should take into consideration the risk of acute complications during treatment and the long-term risk of cancer treatment upon orofacial structures. Acute oral infections during cancer treatment can be difficult to manage, may disrupt therapy, and in patients who are at risk for developing neutropenia, more serious infection and sequelae may ensue. Due to permanent diminished bony healing capacity caused by RT, teeth with poor prognosis resulting from caries and/or periodontal disease in the RT field should be extracted, ideally 2–3 weeks prior to the start of RT to allow for appropriate bony healing (Alert Box 10.1). Untreated caries and periodontal disease should also be managed during

---

Alert Box 10.1 Prevention of oral treatment complications associated with surgical procedures that cause direct osseous Injury.

Prior to treatment with high-potency antiresorptive medications:
Dentoalveolar surgery and/or extraction of teeth with poor prognosis 2–3 weeks prior to initiation of therapy

Patients with ongoing or history of high-potency antiresorptive medications:
Consider alternative treatment to prevent medication-associated ONJ

Prior to RT treatment:
Dentoalveolar surgery and/or extraction of teeth with poor prognosis in planned RT field 2–3 weeks prior to initiation of therapy

Patients with history of RT to the head and neck:
Consider alternative treatment to prevent PRON if planned treatment is in RT field
Consider HBO treatment prior to and after surgical procedure if planned treatment is in RT field

this time to eliminate any potential sources of acute infection and caries progression during treatment and prevent the need for future surgery in radiated sites. Further, potential causes of oral trauma such as sharp tooth edges or ill-fitting dental prostheses should be adjusted to prevent mucosal injury during treatment, and long-term daily utilization of fluoride delivered in custom trays is an important preventive strategy to minimize radiation-associated dental caries.

10.1.2   Hematologic malignancies

Patients with hematologic malignancies often have profoundly compromised immune systems prior to initiation of therapy, are typically treated with multiple courses of high-dose chemotherapy resulting in extended periods of myelosuppression/immunosuppression, and in some cases may be considered for *hematopoietic stem cell transplantation* (HSCT).

Chemotherapy regimens may involve *induction therapy*, in which combined agent chemotherapy is utilized to rapidly obliterate most of the tumor cells to cause the cancer to go into remission, followed by *consolidation chemotherapy*, when high doses of chemotherapeutics serve to further reduce tumor burden. In autologous HSCT, the patient's stem cells are collected prior to intensive myeloablative conditioning (with or without total body irradiation) and then reinfused as a "stem cell rescue" after chemotherapy. Allogeneic HSCT involves either myeloablative or reduced-intensity conditioning followed by infusion of stem cells from a human leukocyte antigen (HLA)-matched donor, which results in restoration of hematopoiesis and immune function, and long-term anticancer therapy through the graft-versus-tumor effect. Intensive chemotherapy regimens place patients at high risk for infection and bleeding (see chapters 3 and 4), and patients undergoing allogeneic HSCT are at significant risk for developing oral chronic graft-versus-host disease and its many sequalae.

Patients scheduled for HSCT should have potential sources of acute infection removed at least 1 week prior to the start of induction CT to allow for soft tissue healing and to assess for resolution of symptoms. This includes extractions of hopeless teeth, endodontic therapy, caries control, periodontal treatment, and dental prophylaxis. Patients may be at risk for infection and/or bleeding following dental procedures secondary to neutropenia and thrombocytopenia, especially surgical procedures or dental scaling. A thorough evaluation of laboratory values, including platelet and absolute neutrophil counts, must be obtained prior to performing dental treatment, and precautions should be taken if necessary (see chapters 3 and 4). Finally, patients should be instructed on meticulous oral hygiene practices and educated about the potential early and late oral effects of cancer treatment.

10.1.3   Antiresorptive therapy

Patients with multiple myeloma and solid cancers that have metastasized to bone may be treated with intravenous (IV) aminobisphosphonate or high-dose denosumab (a receptor activator of nuclear factor kappa-B ligand [RANKL, a potent mediator of bone resorption] inhibitor) therapy to prevent cancer growth and reduce the risk of developing skeletal-related events, such as bone fractures and spinal cord compression. These antiresorptive medications are powerful inhibitors of osteoclastic bone resorption. An untoward side effect of these otherwise very effective treatments is an increased risk of *medication-associated osteonecrosis of the jaw* (ONJ; section 10.4.4).

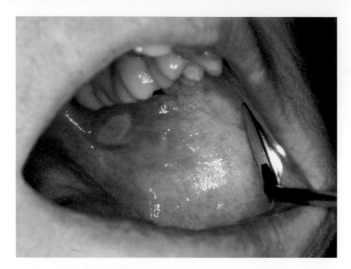

Figure 10.1   Aphthous-like lesion on the left buccal mucosa of a patient on mTOR inhibitor therapy (targeted molecular cancer therapy) for sarcoma management.

Prior to initiation of IV bisphosphonate or high-dose denosumab therapy, non-restorable and hopeless teeth should be extracted and necessary elective dentoalveolar surgery should be completed at least 2–3 weeks prior to treatment to allow for adequate soft tissue and osseous healing (Alert Box 10.1). Further, potential causes of oral trauma such as sharp tooth edges or ill-fitting dental prostheses should be adjusted to prevent mucosal injury. Dental prophylaxes, caries control, and conservative restorative dentistry can be and should be performed while on therapy. For dental management of patients on antiresorptive medications, see section 10.4.4.

10.2   Early effects of cancer treatment

10.2.1   *Surgical procedures*

Acute pain is expected secondary to surgical procedures for head and neck cancer. Surgery-related pain usually involves acute inflammatory responses related to the extent of the surgery and may be associated with a variable degree of concomitant nerve injury. Post-surgical pain is usually self-limiting and is managed with analgesics.

10.2.2   *Oral mucositis*

Oral mucositis is a common acute complication of RT to the head and neck and/or CT. It is a painful and debilitating condition that often results in limited oral intake and weight loss and has a profound effect on quality of life. The increasing use of more aggressive therapy to improve cancer cure rates has increased the frequency, severity, and duration of oral mucositis. In addition, newer anticancer therapies, such as the mTOR inhibitors, are associated with new forms of mucositis that present differently from classic CT- or RT-induced lesions (Figure 10.1).

Oral mucositis generally manifests as erythema followed by ulceration of mucosal tissue (Figure 10.2). Diagnosis is made through clinical examination, and routine assessment of the oral cavity during cancer treatment permits early identification of lesions. In an effort to

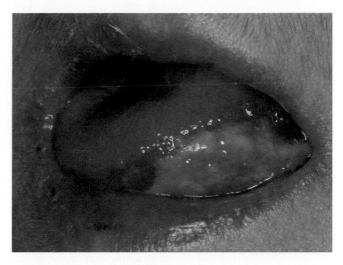

Figure 10.2   Severe mucositis of the left lateral tongue in a patient undergoing chemotherapy and radiotherapy for squamous cell carcinoma of the left lateral tongue.

Grade 0: No oral mucositis
Grade 1: Erythema and soreness
Grade 2: Ulcers, able to eat solids
Grade 3: Ulcers, requires liquid diet (due to mucositis)
Grade 4: Ulcers, alimentation not possible (due to mucositis)

Figure 10.3   World Health Organization Oral Toxicity Scale.
Reference: Sonis ST, Filers JP, Epstein JB, et al. Validation of a new scoring system for the assessment of clinical trial research of oral mucositis induced by radiation or chemotherapy. Mucositis Study Group. Cancer 1999;85(10):2103–2013.

Oral mucositis (functional/symptomatic)
Grade 1: Asymptomatic or mild symptoms; intervention not indicated
Grade 2: Moderate pain; not interfering with oral intake; modified diet indicated
Grade 3: Severe pain; interfering with oral intake
Grade 4: Life-threatening consequences; urgent intervention indicated
Grade 5: Death

Figure 10.4   National Cancer Institute (NCI) Common Toxicity Criteria for Adverse Events (CTCAE) version 4.0.
Reference: Common Toxicity Criteria for Adverse Events v4.0 (CTCAE). Available at: http://evs.nci.nih.gov/; accessed June 15, 2011.

standardize measurements of mucosal integrity, oral assessment scales have been developed to grade the severity and extent of mucositis. The most frequently utilized scales are the World Health Organization Oral Mucositis Scale, which combines subjective and objective measures of oral mucositis (Figure 10.3), and the National Cancer Institute (NCI) Common Terminology Criteria for Adverse Events (CTCAE) version 4.0, a subjective scale used by oncologists in clinical practice to grade treatment-related toxicity (Figure 10.4).

Mucositis typically develops 7–14 days following initiation of CT. While high-dose CT regimens may cause severe mucositis, patient-specific genetic predisposition is also likely a significant factor. CT-induced oral mucositis exclusively affects the non-keratinized mucosa; this distinction is important since ulcers of the keratinized mucosa most likely represent recrudescent HSV infection (see chapter 7). Ulcerative mucositis occurs in approximately 40% of patients receiving standard CT and about three-quarters of patients who receive high-dose CT. Mucositis is self-limiting when uncomplicated by infection and typically heals within 2–4 weeks after cessation of CT.

Radiation-induced oral mucositis is the result of cumulative tissue dose and is almost universal in patients undergoing treatment involving the oral cavity/oropharynx. Unlike CT, radiation damage is anatomically site-specific, and toxicity is localized to irradiated tissue. The degree of damage is dependent on treatment regimen–related factors including type of radiation used, total dose administered, field site, field size/fractionation, and the inclusion of concomitant chemotherapy. Mucositis in RT often escalates at week 3, peaking at week 5 and persisting for weeks with gradual remission of signs and symptoms after completion of therapy. In patients who receive concomitant CT and RT, the severity and duration of mucositis tissue damage is increased.

Treatment for oral mucositis involves meticulous oral hygiene and symptomatic management in a stepped approach beginning with bland rinses, followed by topical anesthetics/analgesics, mucosal coating agents, and then systemic analgesics. Further, new chemical compounds are being developed with a goal of reducing tissue injury associated with cancer treatment. Palifermin is a growth factor that is approved for use in decreasing oral mucositis in HSCT patients who receive high-dose CT. Amifostine is a chemical radio-protector that neutralizes free-radicals and may have the capacity to reduce treatment effects in patients receiving RT and/or CT.

10.2.3   Oral infection

Acute oral infections of the mucosa, dentition/periapices, and periodontium may occur during and following cancer therapy due to exacerbation of latent or prior chronic infection, changes in flora that occur secondary to cancer treatment, or indirect damage to oral structures and tissues. Clinical findings and modalities to aid in the diagnosis of oral infection are addressed in chapter 7.

Bacterial infection may present as localized or systemic infection, especially during myelosuppression secondary to high-dose CT. As the absolute neutrophil count falls below $1,000/mm^3$ (see chapter 4), the incidence and severity of infection increases. Bacterial infections may not present with the usual pain, swelling, and suppuration if the patient is neutropenic, making clinical detection and diagnosis more difficult. All bacterial infection should be treated early and aggressively.

Candidiasis is a common clinical infection of the oropharynx in patients during and following CT and/or RT. A number of variables contribute to its clinical expression, including immunocompromised status, mucosal injury, and salivary flow. While candidiasis may be treated with topical antifungal agents, systemic medications are more effective and are generally preferable during cancer therapy.

Viral infections can cause a variety of clinical findings that range from mild to serious conditions in patients receiving cancer therapy. In most instances, viral infections result from reactivation of latent virus. The severity and impact of these lesions, including risk for systemic dissemination, dramatically increases with increasing immunosuppression. Prophylaxis with antiviral medications for patients receiving high-dose CT and undergoing HSCT has considerably reduced the incidence of herpes simplex virus and cytomegalovirus reactivation.

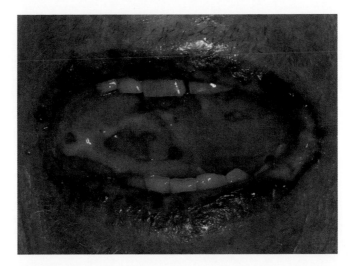

Figure 10.5   55-year-old male at day 60 following allogeneic hematopoietic stem cell transplantation for chronic lymphocytic leukemia. The patient developed acute GVHD with erythema and desquamation of the skin, and oral manifestations included severe intraoral ulcerations with erythema and pseudomembrane formation.

During the first few months following allogeneic HSCT, patients are at increased risk for developing *post-transplant lymphoproliferative disorders* (PTLDs), a diverse group of disorders ranging from benign hyperplasias to malignancies. PTLD has been attributed to proliferation of Epstein-Barr virus (EBV) transformed B-lymphocytes, although EBV-negative disease has been reported in late (greater than 1 year post-transplant) PTLD cases.

10.2.4 *Acute graft-versus-host disease*

Patients who have received allogeneic HSCT are at risk for graft-versus-host disease (GVHD), which is the result of donor cells that react with and destroy host tissue. GVHD may be classified as acute or chronic. Acute GVHD (aGVHD) generally develops within the first 100 days following HSCT but can occur as early as 1 week and as late as over 1 year post-transplantation. Acute GVHD most commonly presents as a pruritic erythematous rash on the skin, followed by involvement of the liver (elevated liver function tests) and gastrointestinal tract (diarrhea). Oral mucosal lesions are less common and may present as erythematous, desquamative, and/or ulcerative lesions (Figure 10.5).

10.3 Early/late effects of cancer treatment

10.3.1 *Hyposalivation*

Ionizing radiation can cause permanent damage to salivary glands that are included in the radiation fields. Irreversible effects occur at total doses of greater than 25 Gy, resulting in inflammatory and degenerative changes of salivary acinar cells, alteration in duct epithelium and fibrosis of the connective tissue. During RT, the serous acini are affected earlier than the mucinous acini, resulting in a thick viscous salivary secretion.

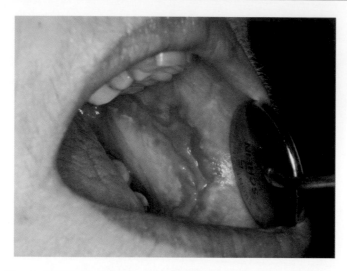

Figure 10.6 Chronic GVHD of the left buccal mucosa, presenting as an ulceration with pseudomembrane formation and surrounding erythema in the center of the lesion. Note the lichenoid appearance with reticular striae affecting the remainder of the buccal mucosa.

Radiation-induced hyposalivation starts early during treatment. In the first week, a 50–60% decrease in salivary flow may occur, and after 7 weeks of conventional RT, salivary flow diminishes to approximately 20%. Following RT, salivary gland function may recover gradually over a 12- to 18-month period. Even when recovery is seen, it is usually incomplete, and reduced salivary flow in such patients is lifelong. Xerostomia, the subjective complaint of a dry mouth, is virtually universal in patients who have undergone RT for head and neck cancer. Studies consistently demonstrate that unstimulated whole salivary flow rates less than 0.1 milliliters/minute are considered indicative of hyposalivation (see chapter 8). Salivary gland hypofunction rarely occurs secondary to CT, but it can be a significant complication for patients with chronic GVHD (see section 10.3.2). Sequelae from hyposalivation include reduced or altered taste (dysgeusia) and difficulties in swallowing (dysphagia), chewing, speaking, and use of an oral prosthesis (see chapter 8).

10.3.2 Chronic GVHD

Chronic GVHD (cGVHD) develops in approximately 50% of patients treated with allogeneic HSCT and is the leading cause of non-relapse-related mortality. Changes can present as early as 100 days after HSCT, and the oral cavity is one of the most frequently affected sites, along with the skin (maculopapular rash), eyes (dry and red), and liver (elevated liver function tests), making oral examination important for cGVHD diagnosis and staging. Clinical changes include mucosal erythema, lichenoid lesions (striae, raised white plaques, patches), ulcerations, and fibrosis (Figure 10.6). Reduced salivary function due to cGVHD involvement of the major and minor salivary glands is common and can contribute to the development of rampant dental decay. Oral symptoms include xerostomia, pain and sensitivity to acidic or spicy foods, alcohols and flavoring agents, especially mint flavors in toothpaste and oral care products.

Diagnosis of oral cGVHD can almost always be made clinically, although in some cases biopsy of the mucosa or minor salivary glands can be helpful for histologic confirmation of the diagnosis.

Management of cGVHD may include topical or systemic steroids and/or immunosuppressive agents as well as management of hyposalivation, secondary oral infections, and increased caries risk. Patients with a history of cGVHD are at significantly increased risk for development of oral cancer (see chapter 9) due to long-term use of immunosuppressants for treatment of cGVHD. Consequently, all patients should be followed regularly and any suspicious lesions should be biopsied.

10.3.3   Neuropathic pain and neurotoxicity

Neuropathic pain is a potentially debilitating form of pain that occurs when peripheral, autonomic and/or central nerves are injured (see chapter 12). Chemotherapeutic agents used for cancer treatment can initiate painful peripheral neuropathies, known as *chemotherapy-induced peripheral neuropathy* (CIPN). Typically, the neuropathic pain is transient, but in some patients may evolve into a chronic pain syndrome resulting in sensory and motor changes that worsens with repeated cycles of chemotherapy. Potentially neurotoxic agents such as the taxanes (paclitaxel, docetaxel), vinca alkaloids (vincristine, vinblastine), platinum-based compounds (cisplatin, oxaliplatin), thalidomide, and bortezamib are most commonly associated with CIPN. Radiation therapy may also cause neural damage resulting in neuropathic pain. Higher total dose regimens and concomitant therapies may contribute to an elevated risk.

Diagnosis is based upon patient self-reports of pain and sensory alteration. Pain is a prominent symptom that typically presents as a paresthesia in the form of unpleasant tingling or burning. Sensory signs include hypersensitivity or decreased sensation to touch, pin, vibration perception, and temperature. Muscle weakness can occur as facial nerve palsy in severe circumstances, and rarely, trismus and slurred speech have been reported. Beyond the orofacial complex, CIPN may develop in the hands and feet, and diagnostic evaluation may include assessment of nerve conduction velocity, electromyography, evoked potential testing, and autonomic testing. Once appropriately diagnosed, management of orofacial neuropathic pain includes a multidisciplinary approach toward pain control and counseling.

10.3.4   Nutrition, taste, and smell impairment

Taste is altered as an early response to RT and may present as a distortion of normal taste (*dysgeusia*), reduction in taste (*hypogeusia*), or an absence of taste sensation (*ageusia*). Taste can also be affected by CT and/or high-dose conditioning prior to HSCT, or due to cGVHD. Taste loss is often noted with radiation doses of 20 Gy, by 30 Gy all taste qualities are affected, and 90% of all patients experience a loss of taste when the cumulative dose has reached 60 Gy, a standard cumulative RT dose. Taste loss appears to be mediated by direct (via RT) or indirect (via CT) damage to the cells in taste buds and/or innervating fibers and is often transient. Damaged cells usually regenerate within 4 months of treatment, so taste returns to normal or near-normal levels within 1 year post-RT or -CT.

Alterations of smell may also develop with RT when the olfactory mucosa is exposed to radiation. This occurs more commonly in the course of treatment for nasopharyngeal carcinoma and maxillary sinus cancers. During RT, smell acuity may be reduced (*hyposmia*) or lost (*anosmia*), or an altered recognition of odor (*dysosmia*) may develop. Similar to taste, smell changes are often transient, and complete recovery often occurs within 1 year following treatment.

Diagnosis of taste and smell impairments is initially made through patient history, though it is important to differentiate between taste and smell changes since the two are related and contribute to the perception of flavor. Diagnosis of a taste disorder begins with questioning the patient about salivation, swallowing, chewing, and oral hygiene. The initial history assessment should also consider contributing systemic diseases beyond cancer treatment, such as diabetes mellitus, hypothyroidism, or gastroesophageal reflux disease. When considering a smell disorder, conditions such as rhinitis, sinusitis, and nasal polyps must first be ruled-out. Physical examination should include assessment of intraoral tissues for local factors that may contribute to taste impairment, such as soft tissue pathology. If a smell disorder is suspected, nasal passages should be evaluated for inflammation, polyps, and obstruction.

To further classify taste dysfunction, regional or whole mouth gustatory testing may be performed (typically at a specialized academic center). For regional testing, small quantities (20–50 microliters) of liquid stimuli are applied to the anterior and posterior tongue using a pipette, soaked filter paper, or cotton-tipped applicator. Whole mouth testing is performed by administering two to ten microliters of solution and asking the patient to swish the solution around in the mouth. Threshold tests for sucrose (sweet), citric acid (sour), sodium chloride (salty), and quinine or caffeine (bitter) are typically compared to natural stimuli, such as pure water. The threshold is the concentration at which the patient correctly identifies the taste three times in a row.

Olfaction dysfunction can be assessed by pressing one nostril shut and placing a vial containing a pungent odor such as coffee, cinnamon, or tobacco under the open nostril, and then repeating the test on the other nostril. If the patient can identify the substance, olfaction is presumed intact. However, this test is crude and sometimes unreliable.

Taste and smell impairments greatly impact the patient's quality of life and, coupled with other RT-related comorbidities such as hyposalivation, dysphagia, and reduced food enjoyment, can adversely affect the nutritional status and overall health of the patient.

10.4   Late effects of cancer treatment

10.4.1   Chronic mucosal changes

The mucosal changes that occur with CT are usually acute, and healing occurs within weeks of cessation of cytotoxic CT. Chronic changes involving oral mucosa are the result of hypovascular, hypocellular, and hypoxic changes that occur following RT. The tissue can become atrophic and friable, especially without the normal lubricating properties of saliva, and may be predisposed to ulceration following minor trauma. Rarely, these changes lead to necrosis of the soft tissue. Fibrosis, or tightening and thickening of the connective tissue, can also occur and may contribute to reduced mobility (Figure 10.7). Additionally, cGVHD can induce chronic mucosal changes such as perioral fibrosis (see section 10.3.2).

10.4.2   Caries

Dental caries risk increases in patients with salivary gland hypofunction following cancer treatment. In addition to hyposalivation, RT and cGVHD can induce alterations in the composition and quality of saliva, which may increase the risk of dental demineralization and caries progression. These alterations include decreased concentration of antimicrobial proteins, reduced remineralizing potential, and loss of buffering capacity. Furthermore, a shift toward a cariogenic flora occurs, as an increased colonization with *Streptococcus mutans* and *lactobacillus* species has been observed in patients who have

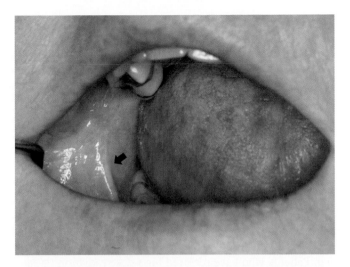

Figure 10.7 Fibrosis of the right buccal mucosa as a chronic mucosal change secondary to radiation therapy for oral squamous cell carcinoma.

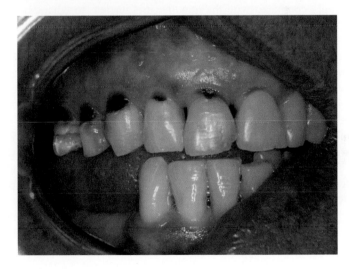

Figure 10.8 Cervical dental caries primarily affecting the cervical portions of maxillary teeth in a patient who underwent radiation treatment for oral squamous cell carcinoma.

undergone RT. Clinically, caries associated with significant hyposalivation affects the interproximal and cervical portions of teeth, and decay is often rampant and progresses quickly (Figure 10.8). Consequently, frequent recall visits at 6-month intervals with appropriate examination and diagnostic radiographs are important for early identification of carious lesions.

To decrease caries risk, optimal oral hygiene must be maintained. Hyposalivation should be managed with systemic cholinergic medications, reinforcing frequent sips of water, and palliated with over-the-counter salivary substitutes and/or stimulants. Caries resistance can be enhanced with use of prescription-strength topical fluorides and/or remineralizing agents that are high in calcium phosphate and fluoride.

10.4.3 Post-radiation osteonecrosis

Post-radiation osteonecrosis (PRON) is another well-recognized complication of head and neck RT. Loss of bone vitality occurs secondary to injury to osteocytes, osteoblasts, and osteoclasts, as well as hypoxia due to reduction in vascular supply. These changes can lead to a reduced healing and regenerative capacity of soft tissue and bone, so that following any type of injury or surgical procedure, the tissue is at risk for developing necrosis. Diagnosis of PRON is made through clinical examination and is defined by the persistence (greater than 2 months) of exposed necrotic bone in the maxilla or mandible (Figures 5.3 and 10.9). Presenting clinical features include symptomatic or asymptomatic exposure of necrotic bone or bone sequestrae, diminished or complete loss of sensation (in most cases unilateral chin paresthesia or anesthesia), and symptoms related to secondary infection, including swelling, tenderness, pain, and fistula formation. In severe cases pathologic fracture may occur.

The risk for PRON is directly related to radiation technique as well as dose and volume of tissue irradiated. Patients who have received high-dose radiation (greater than 60 Gy) to the head and neck are at risk for PRON for life, with an overall risk of approximately 5%. PRON more frequently involves the mandible, likely due to greater bone density and unilateral vascular supply compared with the maxilla. It is unclear to what extent newer radiotherapy techniques, which provide a more focused but locally more intense dose, may or may not affect the incidence of PRON.

Prevention of PRON involves a thorough oral evaluation and removal of unsalvageable teeth prior to initiation of RT (see section 10.1.1, Alert Box 10.1). Management of PRON includes removal of bony sequestrae and use of topical and systemic antimicrobial therapy, which may facilitate wound stabilization and, in some cases, resolution. In cases associated with pain and progression, hyperbaric oxygen therapy (HBO) may be recommended, although the efficacy of this treatment remains unclear. HBO can potentially increase oxygenation of irradiated tissue, promote angiogenesis, and enhance osteoblast repopulation and fibroblast function. Further, preventive HBO therapy may be recommended in patients who require dental extractions or other surgical procedures in areas that have been affected by high-dose RT (Alert Box 10.1).

The literature is inconclusive regarding the safety of dental implant placement following head and neck RT. Patients who have dental implants in the field of radiation may have an increased risk of long-term implant failure.

10.4.4 Medication-associated osteonecrosis of the jaw

Antiresorptive agents such as oral bisphosphonates and low-dose subcutaneous (SQ) denosumab (Priola) are commonly used in the management of osteoporosis (see chapter 5), while high-potency IV bisphosphonates and SQ denosumab (Xgeva) are important agents in cancer treatment, primarily in patients with bone metastases. Clinically, non-healing, exposed, necrotic bone in the maxillofacial region, representing ONJ, has been described in patients treated with antiresorptive medications (Figure 10.10). Further, there have been reports of ONJ associated with *vascular endothelial growth factor* (VEGF) *inhibitors* (e.g., bevacizumab, sunitinib) taken alone or, more frequently, in combination with high-potency antiresorptive medication therapy.

Diagnosis of ONJ is primarily based on patient history and clinical examination. The American Association of Oral and Maxillofacial Surgeons (AAOMS) has established

(a)

(b)

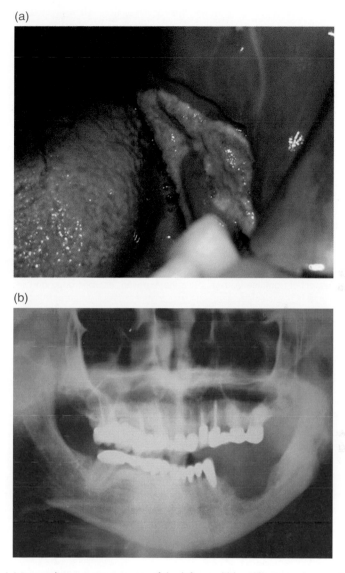

Figure 10.9   (a) Post-radiation osteonecrosis of the left mandible with exposed, necrotic bone; and (b) panoramic radiograph showing loss of cortical bone in the left mandible. Reprinted from Dental Clinics of North America 52(1), Fischer DJ and Epstein JB, Management of patients who have undergone head and neck cancer therapy," pgs. 39–60, 2008, with permission from Elsevier.

a definition of ONJ that is comprised of the following: (1) current or previous treatment with a antiresorptive medication, (2) exposed, necrotic bone in the maxillofacial region that has persisted for more than 8 weeks, and (3) no history of radiation therapy to the jaws. While the epidemiology remains poorly defined, it appears that up to 5% of patients on monthly high-potency antiresorptive agents develop ONJ, with those on oral or low-dose SQ therapy being at a significantly lower risk (0.01–0.34%) and generally developing less severe disease. Exposed, yellow-white, hard bone may vary in size from a few millimeters to a few centimeters and is clinically identical to lesions seen in PRON (Figures 10.9 and 10.10).

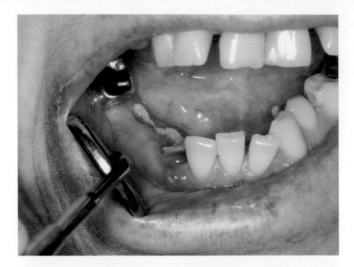

Figure 10.10 Medication-associated ONJ of the right mandible in a patient treated with antiresorptive therapy for management of bony metastases. Note the exposed, necrotic bone and secondary soft tissue infection.

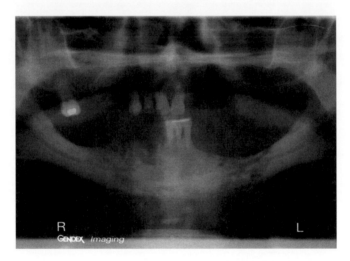

Figure 10.11 Radiographic image illustrating an advanced case of medication-associated ONJ in a 70-year-old male with multiple myeloma on monthly zoledronic acid therapy. Dense sclerotic and mixed mottled (poorly defined radiolucent/radiopaque) changes are affecting the body of the mandible, and persistent extraction sockets are present in the right anterior mandible.

Lesions typically become symptomatic when surrounding tissues become inflamed or secondarily infected, and intraoral or extraoral sinus tracts may develop. Radiographic findings are usually negative with early lesions, although widening of the periodontal ligament space may be seen in dentate patients. Advanced cases may show a moth-eaten, poorly defined mixed radiolucent/radiopaque lesion, a finding that may also occur with PRON lesions or bony malignancies (Figure 10.11). Approximately 50% of cases are associated with a dental extraction or surgical procedure, with the remaining 50% developing spontaneously, often in the lingual mylohyoid ridge area or an exostosis.

Prevention of ONJ involves a thorough oral evaluation and removal of unsalvageable teeth prior to initiation of antiresorptive medication (section 10.1.3, Alert Box 10.1). After high-potency antiresorptive therapy has begun, procedures that involve direct osseous injury should be avoided if reasonable alternative therapies are available (Alert Box 10.1). For example, non-restorable teeth may be treated by removal of the crown and endodontic treatment of the remaining roots. However, persistent chronic infection is a significant risk factor for the development of ONJ; therefore, when necessary, teeth should be expertly extracted with minimal trauma to bone, and in most cases extraction sites heal without complications. There is no evidence that treatment with pre- and/or post-treatment antibiotics or HBO therapy reduces the risk of developing ONJ.

Treatment for ONJ is primarily directed at eliminating or controlling pain, inflammation, and infection, as described above for PRON. In more severe cases of recurrent or prolonged infection, long-term antibiotic therapy is necessary. While surgery may be indicated in severe cases, or when pathologic fracture develops, there is no evidence to date to support the use of HBO therapy or any other non-standard adjunctive treatments.

10.4.5   Trismus and other musculoskeletal presentations

Trismus, defined as a progressive reduction in mouth opening, may develop if the masticatory muscles and/or temporomandibular joint (TMJ) are affected by head and neck cancer treatment. Surgical treatment may produce scar tissue, which reduces mouth opening due to contraction and fibrosis of the masticatory muscles and surrounding myofascia. Additionally, RT may induce fibrosis and atrophy in the masticatory muscles and/or TMJ structures as a late radiation effect if the radiation field involves the TMJ and adjacent musculature. The prevalence of trismus after head and neck cancer treatments ranges from 5% to 38%, is highly unpredictable, and usually develops 3–6 months after RT. Trismus may contribute to morbidity since limitation in opening interferes with oral hygiene, speech, nutritional intake, examination of the oropharynx, and dental treatment. As profound salivary gland hypofunction often accompanies trismus, these patients are at very high risk for developing rampant dental caries.

Other musculoskeletal presentations include limited range of motion and mobility of intraoral, perioral, and cervical musculature. Limited opening secondary to progressive fibrosis of the perioral tissues may occur in patients with the sclerotic form of cGVHD. Further, head and neck cancer patients treated with surgery and/or RT may experience cervical and neck fibrosis and limitations in tongue mobility and mandibular movement. This may result in pain, impaired speech articulation, dysphagia, difficulty with mastication, deviation of the mandible during functional movements, poor control of salivary secretions, and disfigurement.

The objectives in managing trismus and other musculoskeletal deficits are to restore range of mandibular movement and to alleviate pain and dysfunction. Physical therapy exercises to increase mouth opening or range of motion with passive stretching, with or without the use of a professional device, can be beneficial (Figure 10.12). Soft tissue and bone graft procedures and intraoral/extraoral prostheses can restore surgical defects and function. Involvement of other health professionals, such as physical and speech therapists, may be warranted. Treatment typically requires long-term, if not life-long, efforts.

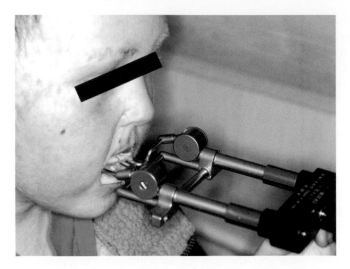

Figure 10.12 10-year-old male post–allogeneic hematopoietic stem cell transplantation with a previous history of severe ulcerative oral chronic GVHD with subsequent peri- and intraoral fibrosis and trismus. This Dynasplint device was utilized to increase range of mandibular movement.

10.4.6 Dentofacial abnormalities

Altered craniofacial and dental growth and development is a frequent complication for children who are long-term cancer survivors after having received CT and/or RT. Developmental disturbances in children treated at younger than 12 years generally affect size, shape, and eruption of teeth as well as craniofacial development. Abnormal tooth formation manifests as decreased crown size, shortened and conical-shaped roots, and microdontia; on occasion, complete agenesis may occur. Eruption of teeth may be delayed, and there is an increased frequency of impacted maxillary canines.

Treatment-related injury to maxillary and mandibular growth centers can compromise full maturation of the craniofacial complex. If bilateral RT is administered, changes tend to be symmetric and the effect is not always clinically evident. When unilateral radiation therapy is provided, asymmetrical changes are usually clinically obvious. When indicated, management typically requires a multidisciplinary team of specialists including oral and maxillofacial surgery, orthodontics, and, in some cases, plastic surgery.

10.4.7 Recurrent disease, second primary cancers, and metastatic disease

Patients treated for head and neck cancers have an increased risk of developing local recurrences and/or second primary cancers. The risk of recurrent disease and/or secondary primary head and neck cancer is dependent upon numerous factors, including tumor size and location, presence of positive lymph nodes upon diagnosis, and risk behaviors such as smoking and human papilloma virus status. Due to the significant risk of developing recurrent disease or a second primary cancer, patients with a history of head and neck cancer must have close surveillance (see chapter 9) and routine follow-up with an oncologist to undergo thorough examination, including flexible laryngoscopy and annual chest x-rays, of all head and neck structures. In the oral cavity, surgery and radiation treatment may induce scar formation and irregular anatomy of structures, thereby complicating evaluation of intraoral tissues.

Metastatic orofacial tumors are rare, though when they occur, the jaw bones are affected more often than the oral soft tissues. Breast, lung, and prostate are the most common solid cancers that metastasize to the jaw bones. Metastatic lesions most commonly occur in the posterior mandible, angle of the jaw, and ramus, and the most common presenting symptoms are pain and paresthesia. Radiographic changes can be radiolucent or radiopaque. The tongue and gingiva are the most common soft tissue sites of metastasis, though pain is a rare complaint in soft tissue metastases.

Patients treated with allogeneic HSCT are at increased risk for developing secondary solid cancers and PTLD (section 10.2.3), and the oral cavity (squamous cell carcinoma) can be a site of initial presentation. A history of cGVHD further increases the risk due to chronic immunosuppressive agents for management of this condition. Since these patients often demonstrate long-term mucosal changes secondary to cGVHD, they must be followed carefully, and any abnormality or area demonstrating significant change, such as a non-healing ulcer of unknown etiology, should be biopsied.

10.5 Selected literature

Brennan MT, Woo SB, Lockhart PB. Dental treatment planning and management in the patient who has cancer. Dent Clin North Am 2008;52(1):19–37.

Common Terminology Criteria for Adverse Events v4.0 (CTCAE). Available at: http://biomedgt.nci.nih.gov/wiki/index.php/Category:CTCAE4 Gastrointestinal disorders, accessed January 3, 2010.

Dahllof G, Heimdahl A, Bolme P, et al. Oral conditions in children treated with bone marrow transplantation. Bone Marrow Transplant 1988;3:43–51.

Dijkstra PU, KIalk WW, Roodenburg JL. Trismus in head and neck oncology: A systematic review. Oral Oncol 2004;40:879–889.

Elad S, Zadik Y, Hewson I, et al. A systematic review of viral infections associated with oral involvement in cancer patients: A spotlight on Herpesviridea. Support Care Cancer 2010;18:993–1006.

Fischer DJ, Epstein JB. Management of patients who have undergone head and neck cancer therapy. Dent Clin North Am 2008;52(1):39–60.

Grangstrom G. Osseointegration in irradiated cancer patients: An analysis with respect to implant failures. J Oral Maxillofac Surg 2005;63(5):579–585.

Hellstein JW, Adler RA, Edwards B, et al. Managing the care of patients receiving antiresorptive therapy for prevention and treatment of osteoporosis: Executive summary of recommendations from the American Dental Association Council on Scientific Affairs. JADA 2011;142:1243–1251.

Hong CHL, Napenas JJ, Hodgson BD, et al. A systematic review of dental disease in patients undergoing cancer therapy. Support Care Cancer 2010;18:1007–1021.

Hovan AJ, Williams PM, Stevenson-Moore P, Wahlin YB, Ohrn KEO, Elting LS, Spijkervet FKL, Brennan MT. A systematic review of dysgeusia induced by cancer therapies. Support Care Cancer 2010;18:1081–1087.

Lowe T, Bhatia S, Somlo G. Second malignancies after allogeneic hematopoietic cell transplantation. Biol Blood Marrow Transplantation 2007;13(10):1121–1134.

Migliorati CA, Woo S-B, Hewson I, et al. A systematic review of bisphosphonate osteonecrosis (BON) in cancer. Support Care Cancer 2010;18:1099–1106.

Ruggiero SL, Ddson TB, Assael LA, et al. American Association of Oral and Maxillofacial Surgeons position paper on bisphosphonate-related osteonecrosis of the jaws—2009 update. J Oral Maxillofac Surg 2009;67(5 Suppl):2–12.

Scully C, Sonis S, Diz PD. Oral mucositis. Oral Dis 2006;12(3):229–241.

Vissink A, Jansma J, Spijkervet FK, et al. Oral sequalae of head and neck radiotherapy. Crit Rev Oral Biol Med 2003;14:199–212.

Woo SB, Hellstein JW, Kalmar JR. Narrative review: Bisphosphonates and osteonecrosis of the jaws. Ann Intern Med 2006;144:753–761.

Yamada H, Chihara J, Hamada K, et al. Immunohistology of skin and oral biopsies in graft-versus-host disease after bone marrow transplantation and cytokine therapy. J Allergy Clin Immunol 1997;100(6 Pt 2):S73–S76.

11 Oral Manifestations of Autoimmune, Immune-Mediated, and Allergic Disorders

11.0 INTRODUCTION

An intact immune system is essential for health, and in the context of oral diseases, is critical for the prevention and clearance of infections. Many disorders are characterized by an exaggerated response of the immune system, producing inflammatory or autoimmune reactions that lead to further disease. These conditions can be broadly classified as autoimmune, immune-mediated, and allergic disorders, each being potentially associated with oral manifestations. Management of these disorders depends largely on the clinical diagnosis and severity of features, and frequently requires topical and/or systemic immunomodulatory therapies for management. Oral health providers should be aware of the potential oral manifestations of these disorders, as they can be associated with significant morbidity and in some cases may be the initial presenting feature of the disease. This chapter will describe the clinical diagnostic features of the most commonly encountered autoimmune, immune-mediated, and allergic disorders with oral manifestations.

11.1 Autoimmune conditions

Autoimmune diseases result from loss of self-tolerance or an overactive immune response and are characterized by the production of circulating autoantibodies and immune complexes. In addition to autoantibody production by plasma cells, T-cells also play an integral and critical role in the pathogenesis of autoimmune conditions. Approximately 5–8% of the U.S. population has been diagnosed with autoimmune disease, and women are more likely than men to be affected. Diagnosis can be challenging due to a myriad of signs and symptoms that can develop over months to years prior to full disease presentation. The etiology of autoimmune disorders is poorly understood, though it is likely associated with genetic, infectious, and/or environmental factors. Some conditions primarily target epithelium, resulting in *vesiculobullous disorders*, while others primarily affect connective tissue and are known as *collagen vascular diseases*. The diagnosis and evaluation of Sjögren syndrome, an autoimmune disease with significant oral considerations, is covered in detail in chapter 8.

Risk Assessment and Oral Diagnostics in Clinical Dentistry, First Edition.
Dena J. Fischer, Nathaniel S. Treister and Andres Pinto.
© 2013 John Wiley & Sons, Inc. Published 2013 by John Wiley & Sons, Inc.

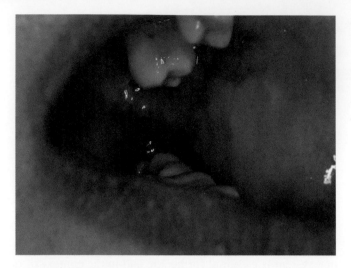

Figure 11.1 Collapsed bulla in a 52-year-old female with pemphigus vulgaris.

11.1.1 *Autoimmune conditions that target epithelium*

11.1.1.1 *Pemphigus vulgaris*

Pemphigus vulgaris (PV) is a rare autoimmune vesiculobullous condition that causes mucosal and cutaneous lesions, with oral involvement often being the first sign of the disease. If left untreated, PV can be life-threatening due to extensive skin ulcerations and infection. The skin lesions appear as blistering eruptions (vesicles or bullae) with a raw erythematous base. Any mucosal and/or skin surface can be involved, including oral as well as conjunctival, pharyngeal, and laryngeal mucosa. Oral vesicles and bullae are rarely observed as they quickly break down, resulting in large, irregular ulcerations (Figure 11.1). During clinical examination of patients with autoimmune vesiculobullous disorders, a blister can be induced secondary to soft tissue manipulation, which is referred to as a positive *Nikolsky sign*.

Pemphigus is characterized by the production of autoantibodies to desmogleins (integral proteins in the desmosomes that confer epithelial cell to cell adhesion), which can be detected in affected tissues (via direct immunofluorescence [DIF]; see chapter 1) as well as in the systemic circulation (via serum-based indirect immunofluorescence [IIF] or enzyme-linked immunosorbent assay [ELISA]). Intact biopsy specimens of pemphigus may reveal intraepithelial separation with preservation of the epithelial basal cell layer, often described as a "row of tombstones." Diagnosis should be confirmed by DIF, which reveals autoantibodies (usually IgG or IgM and complement) in the intercellular spaces between the epithelial cells, resulting in the classic "fishnet" appearance (Figure 11.2). IIF evaluates circulating blood for the presence of specific immunoreactants directed against epithelial structures and may be useful in distinguishing pemphigus from pemphigoid and other oral diseases. In PV, IIF antibody titers correlate to the level of clinical disease and can be useful in assessing response to therapy. Further, autoantibody tests for levels of PV antigens desmogleins 1 and 3 are commercially available and correlate to disease activity in a similar manner as IIF findings.

Paraneoplasic pemphigus is a PV-like disease that occurs infrequently in patients with an underlying neoplasm and/or lymphoproliferative disorder, with the most frequent being non-Hodgkin lymphoma, Castleman disease, chronic lymphocytic leukemia, thymoma, sarcoma, and lung carcinoma. This disorder tends to have a severe and progressive phenotype, with extensive and painful ulcerations primarily affecting the lips, tongue, soft palate, and

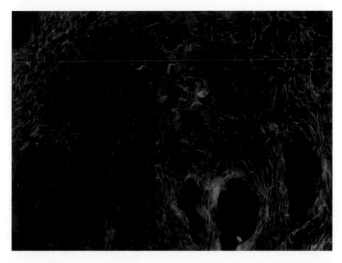

Figure 11.2   Direct immunofluorescence pattern of a tissue specimen from a patient with pemphigus vulgaris.

conjunctiva. Certain drugs like captopril and penicillamine can trigger a PV-like drug hypersensitivity reaction that reverses once the drug is withdrawn.

11.1.1.2   *Pemphigoid*

Mucous membrane pemphigoid (MMP), also known as *cicatricial pemphigoid*, is a vesiculobullous autoimmune disease that affects oral and other mucosal surfaces including conjunctival, nasal, and vaginal mucosa. Skin lesions associated with pemphigoid are characterized by bullae that eventually rupture, followed by crusting and healing without scarring. A significant complication of MMP with ocular involvement is conjunctival scarring (symblepharon) and blindness; therefore all patients diagnosed with pemphigoid require monitoring by an ophthalmologist. Pemphigoid is characterized by autoantibodies directed against hemidesmosomes, which connect the basal epithelium to the basement membrane and the underlying connective tissue, resulting in subepithelial separation and bulla formation. Intact intraoral blisters are observed more frequently compared with PV due to the greater thickness of the blister "roof" (Figure 11.3). Eventually bullae rupture, producing ulcerated lesions that appear clinically similar to those of PV and generally heal without scarring. MMP often presents as a *desquamative gingivitis*, in which the gingival epithelium spontaneously sloughs or can be easily removed with minor manipulation, resulting in erythematous and/or ulcerated gingiva.

Biopsy specimens of pemphigoid demonstrate a split between the epithelium and the underlying connective tissue, with complete separation of the basal epithelium from the basement membrane. DIF shows a continuous linear band of immunoreactants (usually IgG and C3) directed at the basement membrane zone (Figure 11.4). IIF for pemphigoid is of limited diagnostic value since circulating antibodies in serum are not consistently present and titers do not correlate with disease activity.

11.1.2   *Autoimmune conditions that target connective tissue*

11.1.2.1   *Lupus erythematosus*

Lupus erythematosus (LE) is the most common autoimmune connective tissue disorder and has a wide spectrum of disease presentation mediated by the deposition of immune

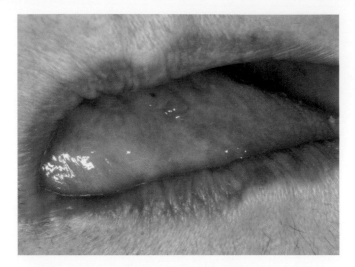

Figure 11.3 Intact bulla on the left lateral tongue of 67-year-old female with mucous membrane pemphigoid complaining of persistent oral soreness.

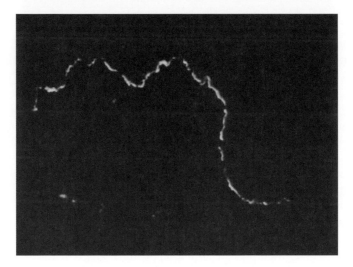

Figure 11.4 Direct immunofluorescence pattern of a tissue specimen from a patient with mucous membrane pemphigoid.

complexes into various organs. Systemic lupus erythematosus (SLE) is a multisystem disease characterized by a cutaneous rash of the malar region secondary to sun exposure (with a "butterfly" appearance; Figure 11.5), renal dysfunction, musculoskeletal manifestations (arthritis and myalgias), cardiac complications (vasculitis, pericarditis, or non-bacterial endocarditis with vegetations affecting the heart valves, termed *Libman-Sacks endocarditis*), and thrombocytopenia (Table 11.1). Oral involvement develops in up to 25% of patients and may present as areas of lichenoid inflammation (section 11.2.2) or non-specific ulcerations that clinically resemble other common oral ulcerative conditions (i.e., recurrent aphthous ulcerations; Table 11.2).

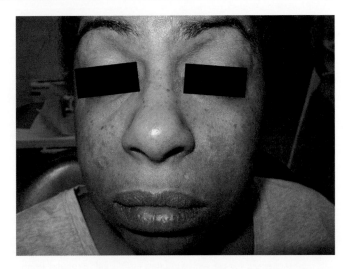

Figure 11.5   Malar rash on the cheeks of a 53-year-old female with systemic lupus erythematosus.

Table 11.1   American College of Rheumatology criteria for classification of systemic lupus erythematosus.*

Presence of 4 or more symptoms simultaneously or serially on two separate occasions

Sign/Symptom	Definition
Malar rash	Rash on cheeks
Discoid rash	Red, scaly patches on skin that cause scarring
Photosensitivity	Exposure to ultraviolet light causes rash or other symptoms of SLE flare-ups
Oral or nasal ulcers	Presence of oral or nasopharyngeal ulcerations
Arthritis	Non-erosive arthritis of two or more peripheral joints, with tenderness, swelling, or effusion
Serositis	Pleurisy (inflammation of the membrane around the lungs) or pericarditis (inflammation of the membrane around the heart)
Serology	≥ 1 of the following in the absence of offending drug: – Hemolytic anemia – Leukopenia (WBC < 4,000 cells/μL) – Lymphopenia (< 1,500 cells/μL) – Thrombocytopenia (< 100,000 cells/μL)
Antinuclear antibody test	Positivity (titer ≥ 1:160)
Immunologic disorder	Positive anti-Smith, anti-ds DNA, antiphospholipid antibody, or positive test result for lupus anticoagulant test using a standard method; or false-positive serologic test for syphilis
Renal disorder	Proteinuria or cellular cases seen in urine microscopically
Neurologic disorder	Seizures or psychosis in the absence of offending drugs

*Modified from http://www.rheumatology.org/practice/clinical/classification/SLE/1997_update_of_the_1982_acr_ revised_criteria_for_classification_of_sle.pdf, accessed February 28, 2012.

Chronic cutaneous lupus erythematosus (CCLE) or *discoid lupus* is a variant of LE in which lesions are generally limited to skin and mucosal surfaces with few or no systemic signs. Skin lesions are characterized by scaly, erythematous patches that typically present on sun-exposed skin surfaces, and healing may result in scarring and hypo- or hyperpigmentation.

Table 11.2   Clinical and laboratory findings of autoimmune, immune-mediated, and allergic conditions with oral manifestations.

Disease	Clinical Presentation	Laboratory Findings
Autoimmune Disease		
Pemphigus vulgaris	Intraepithelial bullae Denuded mucosae/ulcers	LM: intraepithelial separation DIF: antibodies in intercellular spaces (fishnet appearance) IIF: circulating antibodies, correlates with disease activity
Mucous membrane pemphigoid	Subepithelial bullae Desquamative gingivitis Oral ulcers Symblepharon (cicatricial pemphigoid)	LM: subepithelial separation DIF: linear band of IgG, C3 antibodies at basement membrane zone IIF: limited diagnostic utility
Lupus erythematosus	Malar rash Non-specific ulcerations OR lichenoid lesions with radiating striae SLE associated with multisystem complications	LM: subepithelial and perivascular inflammatory infiltrate DIF: granular band of antibodies at basement membrane zone (lupus band test) Serum: elevated ANA (non-specific); anti-DS DNA, anti-Smith (highly specific)
Systemic sclerosis	Raynaud phenomenon Sclerodactyly, fingertip ulcerations Microstomia Widening of periodontal ligament space Loss of gingival attachment Resorption of ramus, condyle, coronoid process Fibrosis of skin and internal organs	LM: accumulation of diffuse fibrotic collagen Serum: elevated ANA, anti-SCL 70 (non-specific)
Rheumatoid arthritis	Bilateral condylar flattening with irregular surface features Inflammatory destruction of joints	Serum: elevated RF, ANA (non-specific); anti-ccp (highly specific)
Mixed connective tissue disease	Overlapping features of SLE, PSS, RA	Serum: elevated ANA (non-specific); anti-IU snRNP (highly specific)
Sjögren syndrome	Salivary hypofunction Dry eyes Joint pain Oral ulceration/pain Dental caries	LM: periductal lymphocytic infiltrate and acini destruction Serum: elevated ANA (non-specific); anti-SSA, anti-SSB (highly specific)
Immune-Mediated Disease		
Lichen planus	Wickham striae Desquamative gingivitis May become erosive, with shallow ulceration	LM: presence of sawtooth rete pegs, subepithelial T-cell infiltrate DIF: subbasement membrane accumulation of fibrinogen
Recurrent aphthous stomatitis	Shallow round or ovoid ulcers with erythematous halo, on non-keratinized mucosa	LM: inflammation (non-specific) Serum: iron, vitamin B_{12}, folate deficiency (associated very rarely)

(Continued)

Table 11.2 (Cont'd)

Disease	Clinical Presentation	Laboratory Findings
Erythema multiforme	Target skin lesions Oral erosions exclude the gingiva Lip crusting	LM: lymphocytes and histiocytes in superficial dermis, leukocyte exocytosis (non-specific)
Inflammatory bowel disease	Cobblestone, linear ulceration Pyostomatitis vegetans Aphthous ulcers Orofacial granulomatosis Angular cheilitis	LM: neutrophil infiltrate in lamina propria, granulomatous inflammation DIF: immune reactivity to IgG, IgM, IgA
Orofacial granulomatosis	Recurrent facial swelling, including the lips and buccal mucosa	LM: edema in lamina propria, granulomatous inflammation (non-caseating), lymphocytic infiltrate
Wegener granulomatosis	"Strawberry" gingivitis Oral ulceration	LM: granulation tissue, eosinophils, multinucleated giant cells IIF: pANCA, cANCA (highly specific) Serum: elevated erythrocyte sedimentation rate, c-reactive protein (non-specific)
Sarcoidosis	Submucosal modules Bilateral parotid swelling Erythematous macules	LM: epitheloid non-caseating granulomas Serum: elevated ACE, serum calcium (non-specific)

Allergic Disorders

Disease	Clinical Presentation	Laboratory Findings
Oral allergy syndrome	Burning, itching, swelling of the mucosa and/or oropharynx	LM: not specific Serum: elevated IgE
Intraoral contact hypersensitivity	Erythema, erosion, edema, pruritus, mucosal lichenoid findings	LM: atrophic or ulcerated epithelium, occasional perivascular lymphoid infiltration, chronic inflammatory infiltrate in lamina propria
Plasma cell gingivitis	Irregular stippling, generalized gingival erythema and edema	LM: dense infiltrate of plasma cells in subepithelial connective tissue
Angioedema	Dermatologic or mucosal edema, itching Respiratory mucosa	LM: not specific Serum: elevated IgE, low (C1-INH)

ACE = angiotensin-converting enzyme
ANA = antinuclear antibody
Anti-ccp = anti–cyclic citrullinated peptide antibody
Anti-DS DNA = anti–double stranded DNA antibody
Anti-IU snRNP = anti–IU small nuclear ribonucleoprotein antibody
Anti-SCL 70 = anti-scleroderma 70 antibody
cANCA = cytoplasmic antineutrophhil cytoplasmic antibody
DIF = direct immunofluorescence
ESR = erythrocyte sedimentation rate
IIF = indirect immunofluorescence
LM = light microscopy
pANCA = perinuclear antineutrophil cytoplasmic antibodies
RF = rheumatoid factor

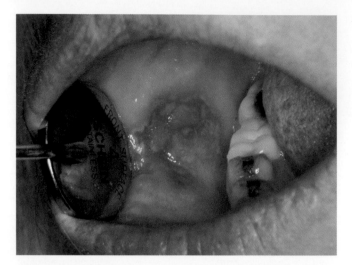

Figure 11.6 Systemic lupus erythematosus lesion on the right buccal mucosa of a young female with an acute flare of symptoms. Note the central erosive presentation with radiating striae.

Oral manifestations of CCLE include classic lichenoid lesions, with characteristic erosions surrounded by white, radiating striae (Figure 11.6).

Lichenoid oral lesions associated with LE may be distinguished from other conditions by the presence of patchy deposits of a periodic acid-Schiff (PAS)-positive material in the basement membrane zone and a subepithelial and perivascular inflammatory infiltrate. DIF shows deposition of immunoreactants (usually IgM, IgG, or C3) in a shaggy or granular band at the basement membrane zone, known as the lupus band test.

Evaluation of serum obtained from a patient with SLE can demonstrate numerous immunologic abnormalities. Most patients (at least 95%) are antinuclear antibody (ANA) positive, a non-specific finding that may also be seen in other autoimmune diseases. In addition, moderate to high titers of anti–double-stranded DNA antibodies are present in 50–60% of patients with SLE, and 30% show anti-Smith antibodies, findings that are highly specific for SLE. Other antibodies highly specific for SLE but found in a relatively small percentage of patients are anti-ribosomal P and antinuclear ribonucleoprotein. Antibodies classically associated with Sjögren syndrome, anti-Ro/SS-A, and anti-La/SS-B may also be present in SLE (Table 11.3; see chapter 8).

11.1.2.2 *Systemic sclerosis*
Systemic sclerosis, also known as *scleroderma*, is a rare autoimmune condition characterized by fibrosis and thickening of body tissues, affecting the skin and internal organs. The two main forms are *progressive systemic sclerosis* (PSS) and *localized scleroderma*. PSS is further divided into *limited cutaneous scleroderma* (previously called CREST syndrome, an acronym for the disease presentation of calcinosis cutis, Raynaud phenomenon, esophageal dysfunction, sclerodactyly, and telangiectasia) and *diffuse cutaneous scleroderma*. Limited cutaneous scleroderma patients often have a history of *Raynaud phenomenon* (vasoconstriction resulting in blanching of the fingertips, usually in cold temperatures), skin sclerosis of the hands resulting in *sclerodactyly* (fibrosis of phalanges resulting in permanent flexure and a "claw-like" appearance, sometimes associated with ulceration of fingertips [Figure 11.7]), esophageal dysmotility resulting

Table 11.3   Important serology values for rheumatologic disorders.

Test	Normal values	Clinical significance
Antinuclear antibodies (ANA)	Titer < 1:160	If titer ≥ 1:160, supportive of autoimmune disease
Anti dsDNA	Titer ≤1:10	If titer > 1:10, supportive of SLE
Anti-Smith	Negative*	If positive, supportive of SLE
SCL-70	Negative*	If positive, supportive of scleroderma
cANCA, pANCA	Titer < 1:80	If titer ≥ 1:80, supportive of Wegener granulomatosis
Ant-ccp	< 20 EU	If > 20 EU, supportive of rheumatoid arthritis
Anti-IU snRNP	< 29 AU 30–40 AU, equivocal	If ≥ 40 AU, supportive of MCTD
Angiotensin-converting enzyme (ACE) levels	8–53 units/L	> 53 units/L, supportive of sarcoidosis
Anti-SSA, Anti-SSB	< 20 units/mL*	> 25 units/mL of either is one criterion for Sjögren syndrome
Rheumatoid factor (RF)	< 30 units/mL	If > 30 U, supportive of autoimmune disease
Erythrocyte sedimentation rate (ESR)	male: age/2 in mm/hr female: (age + 10)/2 in mm/hr	If > 30 mm/hr, non-specific inflammation, may be associated with autoimmune disease

*Quantification units vary depending on laboratory. Results reported as positive or negative.

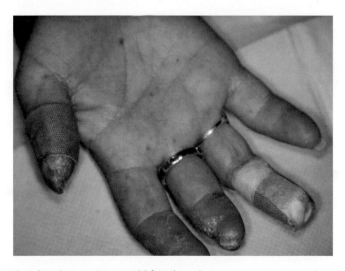

Figure 11.7   Sclerodactyly in a 52-year-old female with progressive systemic sclerosis who presented for consultation regarding facial pain and oral hygiene issues.

from fibrosis of the esophageal submucosa, and calcinosis cutis, manifesting as multiple movable, non-tender subcutaneous nodules.

Diffuse cutaneous scleroderma patients develop widespread skin sclerosis, fibrosis of internal organs, and potentially life-threatening organ failure. Fibrosis of connective tissue in

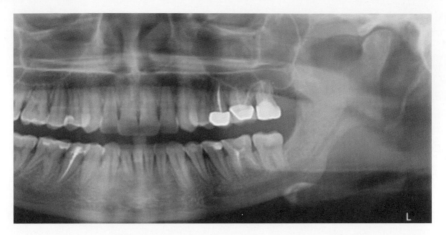

Figure 11.8 Significant mandibular angular notching/resorption in a patient with progressive systemic sclerosis affecting the facial skin.

organs ultimately leads to organ compromise and is most apparent in the lungs, presenting as pulmonary fibrosis, which usually leads to death secondary to cardiac and renal failure. *Localized scleroderma* primarily affects the skin with minimal additional systemic features.

Oral manifestations include microstomia due to sclerosis of perioral tissues, loss of attached gingival mucosa, diffuse widening of the periodontal ligament space, resorption (notching) of the posterior ramus of the mandible and/or condylar heads or coronoid process (Figure 11.8), and fibrosis and rigidity of the tongue, making speaking and swallowing difficult. Secondary Sjögren syndrome is common in patients with scleroderma, and limitations in manual dexterity and/or mouth opening further compound the increased caries risk.

In the serum of patients with systemic sclerosis, ANAs are usually present (more than 90%), and anti-Scleroderma 70 antibodies may also be detected. Because serology is not very specific for the disease, diagnosis of systemic sclerosis is made from the presence of clinical characteristics, particularly cutaneous skin fibrosis with Raynaud phenomenon.

11.1.2.3 *Rheumatoid arthritis*
Rheumatoid arthritis (RA) is an autoimmune disorder characterized by bilateral synovitis and inflammatory destruction and deformation of the joints. Signs and symptoms typically become more severe over time and include swelling, stiffness, pain, joint deformity, and disability, with periods of exacerbation and remission (Figure 11.9). Partially movable, non-tender *rheumatoid nodules* (fibrous tissue covering an area of fibrinoid necrosis) may develop beneath the skin near affected joints. The temporomandibular joints are affected in up to 75% of patients, with symptoms of pain and dysfunction and radiographic features including a flattened condylar head with irregular surface features without loss of joint space (Figure 11.10).

Serology may contribute to diagnosis since approximately 80% of patients with RA exhibit elevated rheumatoid factor (RF), and 50% of patients have elevated ANAs. During active phases of the disease, patients usually exhibit an elevated erythrocyte sedimentation rate (ESR).

11.1.2.4 *Mixed connective tissue disease*
Mixed connective tissue disease (MCTD) is a condition that has overlapping clinical features of SLE, PSS, and/or RA, and there is controversy as to whether it is a distinct clinical

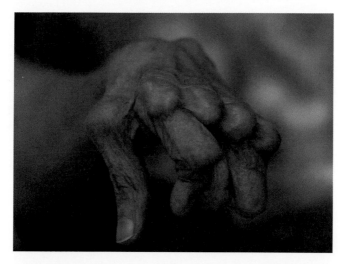

Figure 11.9   Hand deformities in a female with chronic rheumatoid arthritis.

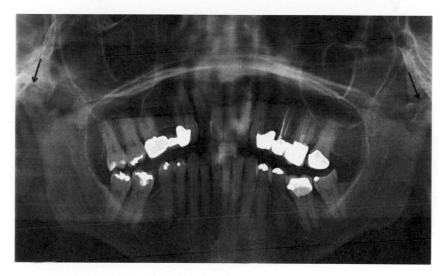

Figure 11.10   Bilateral condylar flattening in a 68-year-old female with rheumatoid arthritis and a maximal interincisal opening of 22 millimeters.

entity. Little has been reported on the oral manifestations of MCTD. Serology for the diagnosis of MCTD requires the presence of anti-IU small nuclear ribonucleoprotein (IU-snRNP) antibodies. High titers of ANAs are also commonly found in the serum of MCTD patients.

11.2   Immune-mediated conditions

Immune-mediated disorders largely resemble autoimmune disorders except that there is an absence of autoantibody production. Despite the lack of autoantibodies, immune-mediated disorders are similarly characterized by a chronic, multisystem inflammatory response with autoreactive clinical features. Immune-mediated disorders may have oral manifestations,

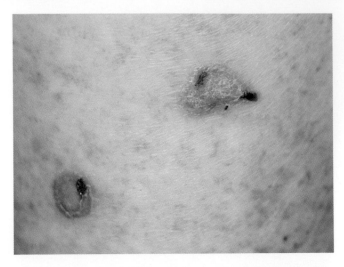

Figure 11.11 Cutaneous lichen planus of the lower leg in a 5-year-old female with concurrent extensive oral involvement. Note the fine striations that appear similar to the classic oral reticular lesions.

which in some cases may be the only feature of the disease, or in other cases may be associated with dermatologic or other systemic manifestations.

11.2.1 Lichen planus

Lichen planus (LP) is a common mucocutaneous condition with prominent oral and dermatologic manifestations. The etiology of LP is largely idiopathic and is believed to be an immune-mediated hypersensitivity response to unknown factors, although medications may be implicated in some cases (section 11.2.2). Cutaneous LP lesions typically present as pruritic papular erythematous-purple scaly rashes with distinct sharp borders and occasional striae (Figure 11.11). Fingernails and genital areas may also be affected. The immune response in LP is mediated by a T-cell reaction to target tissues, with histopathologic findings including a characteristic subepithelial band-like infiltrate of T-lymphocytes and sawtooth rete ridges (epithelial extensions into connective tissue). DIF findings are non-specific and include sub-basement membrane deposition of fibrinogen.

The clinical features of oral LP can be classified as reticular or erosive/erythematous. This classification represents a spectrum of disease presentation, generally corresponding to increasing severity and symptoms. Reticular LP is defined by the presence of reticular striations termed *Wickham striae*, which appear as white, interlacing spider web-like lesions that are generally bilateral and may present on any intraoral keratinized or non-keratinized mucosal surface (Figure 11.12). Erosive LP is characterized by the presence of irregular shallow ulcers of the oral mucosa, often associated with the presence of erythema and reticulation. The most frequently affected sites include the buccal mucosae with extension into the mandibular vestibule and ventrolateral tongue. Gingival involvement is also common and may present as desquamative gingivitis with inflammation of the unattached and attached gingival tissue. The diagnosis of LP can often be made by the distinctive clinical findings alone, although biopsy may be warranted to confirm a diagnosis and/or differentiate between LP and similarly presenting disease. All LP patients should be monitored for mucosal abnormalities given that there is a 1% risk for malignant transformation to squamous cell carcinoma.

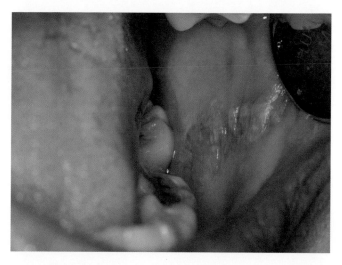

Figure 11.12   Reticular oral lichen planus on the left buccal mucosa of a 33-year-old female.

11.2.2   *Lichenoid reactions*

Lichenoid reactions are delayed-type hypersensitivity responses to an antigen in the superficial layers of the mucosa. Clinically and histologically, lichenoid reactions closely resemble lichen planus, although contact reactions may present with unilateral features localized to a specific mucosal surface. Potential causes of lichenoid reactions include restorative materials in direct contact with the lesion(s), as well as cinnamon, mint, spices, or coloring agents found in food additives. Identification and removal of common allergens often results in resolution of the area and confirms the diagnosis.

The use of medications has also been associated with the onset of lichenoid reactions, with the most common being angiotensin-converting enzyme (ACE) inhibitors, diuretics, non-steroidal anti-inflammatory medications, and beta-blocking agents. The potential association between medication intake and onset of lichenoid reactions is based on a temporal association between the start of the prescription and the onset of disease signs; however, the response can be delayed.

11.2.3   *Recurrent aphthous stomatitis*

Recurrent aphthous stomatitis (RAS) is a condition characterized by recurrent oral ulcerations that affects approximately one-fifth of the population. Lesions appear as shallow round or ovoid ulcerations with a characteristic whitish-gray appearance surrounded by an erythematous halo, primarily affecting non-keratinized mucosa (Figure 11.13). Minor RAS ulcers are less than 1 centimeter in diameter and heal within 1–2 weeks without scarring. In major RAS, the ulcerations are at least 1 centimeter in diameter, can have irregular borders, and can persist for weeks, in some cases with scar formation. Herpetiform RAS can be seen in association with both minor and major RAS and resembles the ulceration patterns seen in human herpesvirus infections (multiple small punctate ulcers that coalesce) but is not of viral etiology. Severe/complex RAS is a potentially debilitating condition that is characterized by nearly continuous and often multiple ulcers, such that patients experience minimal, if any, ulcer-free periods. The etiology of RAS is not well understood but appears to be

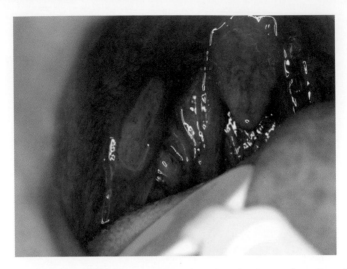

Figure 11.13 Recurrent major aphthous stomatitis in the right soft palate and tonsillar pillar of a 24-year-old male.

related to dysfunction in cytokine production and a hyperactive mucosal immune response. A presumptive association has been proposed between RAS and iron-, vitamin B12- or folic acid–deficiency anemia, albeit a causal relationship is unclear.

There are several other conditions in which RAS is a prominent feature. Behçet disease is a multisystem immune-mediated condition characterized by oral and genital aphthous ulcers, ocular inflammation, and a variety of other features. Oral ulceration can be the presenting sign of the disease. Patients with inflammatory bowel disease, and in particular Crohn disease, may present with severe RAS. Mammalian target of rapamycin (mTOR) inhibitors (e.g., sirolimus), used for both immunosuppressive and antineoplastic activities, are also associated with the development of oral aphthous-like ulcerations (see chapter 10).

Diagnosis of RAS is based on history and the classic clinical presentation. While biopsies may be performed in suspected RAS, histopathology demonstrates non-specific inflammatory findings with a dense T-cell infiltrate. RAS should not be confused with intraoral recrudescent herpes simplex virus (HSV) infection (see chapter 7).

11.2.4 *Erythema multiforme*

Erythema multiforme (EM) is an acute, self-limiting but potentially recurrent, immune-mediated mucocutaneous disorder that is characterized by target-shaped skin lesions, crusting of the lips, and non-specific oral ulcerations (Figure 11.14). EM is often idiopathic but can be triggered by infection (e.g., recrudescent HSV or mycoplasma infections) and drug reactions (e.g., non-steroidal anti-inflammatories, antibiotics). Constitutional symptoms such as fever and lymphadenopathy may also occur, often as a prodrome. EM is classified as EM minor and EM major, depending on the extent and severity of the lesions. EM minor typically presents with a target-like rash eruption on flexor areas, usually in the extremities, without oral involvement. EM major is characterized by perioral and oral involvement in addition to the cutaneous rash. Oral ulcerations may be large and confluent but are largely limited to the non-keratinized mucosa of the anterior oral cavity with sparing of the gingiva, hard palate, and soft palate. Crusting and bleeding of the lips is a common presenting sign

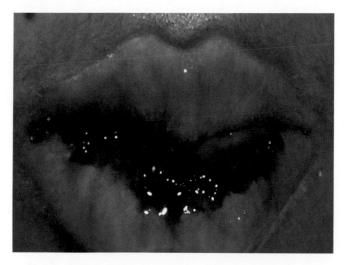

Figure 11.14   Erythema multiforme with lip crusting in a 28-year-old female.

of EM major and is a significant risk factor for nutritional compromise and dehydration. Of note, EM major can be limited to the oral cavity and lips without skin lesions.

EM should not be confused with Stevens-Johnson syndrome or toxic epidermal necrolysis, which are mucocutaneous reactions that may develop as hypersensitivity responses to drugs or infection and can be life-threatening. Cases of recurrent EM that are known to be related to recrudescent HSV (i.e., patient develops herpes labialis and EM develops 1–2 weeks later) can be prevented with prophylactic systemic antiviral treatment.

11.2.5   Granulomatous conditions

Granulomatous conditions encompass several disorders that develop idiopathically or in response to infectious agents, irritation, or foreign bodies. They demonstrate granulomatous inflammation, which is characterized by the presence of multinucleated giant cells, histiocytes, and an intense lymphocytic infiltrate. Several granulomatous conditions are associated with or characterized by prominent orofacial features.

11.2.5.1   *Inflammatory bowel disease*
Crohn disease (CD) and ulcerative colitis (UC) are collectively known as inflammatory bowel diseases (IBDs). They are immune-mediated inflammatory conditions that primarily affect the small and large intestines and are characterized by severe inflammation of the intestine or colon. The oral cavity, as an extension of the gastrointestinal (GI) tract, may also be affected. Of note, oral and GI disease activity do not always correlate, such that oral manifestations may be present when the lower GI symptoms are otherwise stable or in remission.

Oral features may include linear fissure-like ulcerations, a cobblestone appearance of the buccal and labial mucosa, and/or orofacial granulomatosis (section 11.2.5.2). Biopsy specimens of these oral conditions typically demonstrate granulomatous inflammatory changes similar to those seen in the lower GI tract. RAS is a common oral manifestation of CD and sometimes UC, with the severe/complex presentation being encountered more frequently. Angular cheilitis is also a common occurrence (see chapter 7).

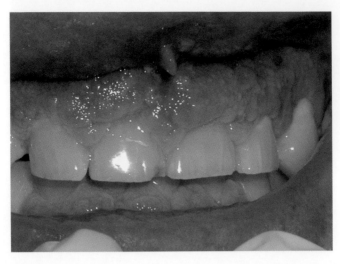

Figure 11.15 Pyostomatitis vegetans in a 37-year-old male with an acute flare of ulcerative colitis complaining of gastrointestinal discomfort.

Pyostomatitis vegetans is a rare oral condition associated with IBD that presents as multiple linear exophytic suppurative lesions, which appear like "snail tracks" primarily observed on the buccal and labial mucosae (Figure 11.15). Biopsy specimens demonstrate a dense infiltrate of neutrophils in the lamina propria and multiple microabscesses, while DIF shows a pericellular pattern with immunoreactants against IgG, IgM, or IgA in a pattern identical to that seen in PV.

A history of GI symptoms should be obtained when any of these oral features are encountered in a patient, as oral findings may be the initial presenting sign or may represent a flare in symptoms or lack of response to therapy.

11.2.5.2 *Orofacial granulomatosis*
Orofacial granulomatosis is a rare disorder characterized by recurrent swelling of the lips and/or buccal mucosa or of the generalized facial tissues (Figure 11.16). In some individuals, swelling episodes can be associated with certain foods and preservatives such as cinnamon, monosodium glutamate, and benzoate, although it can be very difficult to determine the etiology, and restrictive diets are often ineffective. Lesions are typically asymptomatic but can be disfiguring and have a significant psychosocial impact on the patient.

11.2.5.3 *Wegener granulomatosis*
Wegener granulomatosis (antineutrophil cytoplasmic antibodies [ANCA]-associated granulomatous vasculitis, granulomatosis with polyangitis [GPA]) is a rare vasculitic disease that is typically localized to the lungs and kidneys. Oral manifestations include mucosal and gingival erythematous proliferations, also termed "strawberry gingivitis," and ulcerations that can lead to progressive loss of tissue (i.e., of the palate, periodontal supporting structures, and/or nasal cavity; Figure 11.17). The etiology of the disease is unknown.

Diagnosis of Wegener granulomatosis relies on both laboratory testing and tissue biopsy. Elevated levels of perinuclear ANCA (pANCA) and cytoplasmic ANCA (cANCA) are detected using IIF in over 90% of cases. In addition, ESR and C-reactive protein are usually elevated; serum albumin and total protein are often decreased. Patients may also present

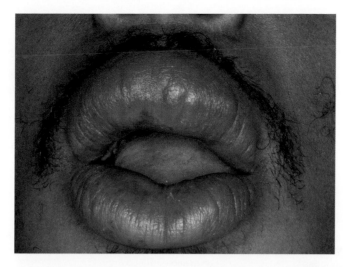

Figure 11.16 Crohn disease presenting as orofacial granulomatosis of the lips in a male with a 10-year history of the disease.

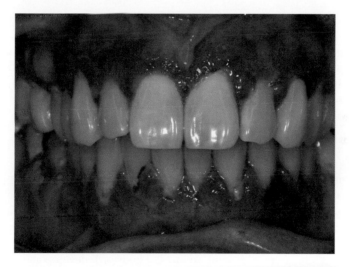

Figure 11.17 Multiple gingival vegetative/granulomatous lesions in a 34-year-old female diagnosed with Wegener granulomatosis.

with anemia and/or thrombocythemia. Histopathologically, biopsy specimens demonstrate granulomatous vasculitis with numerous eosinophils.

11.2.5.4 *Sarcoidosis*

Sarcoidosis is a systemic granulomatous disease of unknown etiology that tends to affect the lungs and lymphatic tissue, although any organ can be involved. The salivary glands are involved in approximately 15% of cases, characterized by bilateral parotid swelling and xerostomia (see chapter 8). Oral mucosal lesions can present as areas of asymptomatic focal granular and erythematous macules that may be associated with submucosal nodules. Cutaneous lesions have a similar clinical presentation to oral lesions.

Table 11.4 Types of allergic reactions.

	Mediators	Characteristics	Clinical Examples
Type I	Histamine, prostaglandin mediators, and leukotrienes	Immediate response, vasodilation, increased vascular permeability	Anaphylaxis, bronchospasm
Type II	Complement, IgG antibodies against cell surface receptors	Slower onset (hours), similar characteristics to type I: increased vascular permeability and vasodilation	Transfusion reaction, acute transplant rejection, hemolytic anemia
Type III	Complement activation by tissue deposition of small immune complexes	May take hours, days, or weeks to develop, presence of acute vascular and renal inflammatory response	Rheumatoid arthritis, glomerulonephritis in SLE, vasculitis
Type IV	Delayed response, sensitized T-lymphocytic activation of macrophages	Takes 2 or 3 days to develop, presence of erythema and mucosal inflammation	Metal or cosmetic contact hypersensitivity, poison ivy

Diagnosis of sarcoidosis relies on blood tests, imaging, and histopathology. Serum ACE levels and calcium levels may be elevated, although neither finding is specific for the disease. Pulmonary hilar adenopathy can be observed in plain chest films and is considered a hallmark of the disease since up to 90% of patients have pulmonary involvement. Minor salivary gland biopsy specimens (even in the absence of clinical salivary gland involvement) may reveal non-caseating granulomas and can contribute to the diagnosis.

11.3 Allergic disorders

Allergic reactions are exaggerated immune responses that may result in host injury. Allergies are often diagnosed in childhood, when individuals are initially exposed to allergens, and children may be more susceptible to develop these reactions due to their maturing immune systems. Many factors play a role in the development of allergic reactions, including genetics, environmental pollutants, and geographic distribution.

Sensitization is a process that involves presentation of an antigen to the immune system and "conditioning" the immune system, so that the body will develop an immune response following re-exposure. Sensitization may be desirable, as occurs in the delivery of vaccines, in which the immune response results in establishment of memory B-cells that subsequently produce a rapid immune response when re-exposed to the pathogen. Alternatively, sensitization may instead lead to development of hypersensitivity, which is an undesirable response after second exposure to an antigen. Hypersensitivity reactions are classified into four types and are associated with a wide range of clinical conditions (Table 11.4).

Testing for allergy to specific materials is done by using "patch tests," in which the suspected antigen is placed in prolonged contact with the patient's skin (usually taped to skin on the back for days). After removal of the material, the local dermatologic response is evaluated (this tests mostly type IV hypersensitivity). An area of severe erythema is considered positive for an allergic response. Of note, patch testing of the skin for potential oral mucosa allergens is generally unreliable, and the significance of positive findings can be unclear and may lead to unnecessary avoidance of certain foods and products.

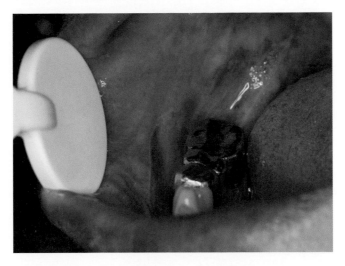

Figure 11.18 Lichenoid response to a metal fixed partial denture on the lower left mandible in a 57-year-old female.

Oral manifestations of allergic disorders include oral allergy syndrome, contact hypersensitivity, plasma cell gingivitis, and angioedema. Orofacial granulomatosis, which is considered by some to be an allergic disorder, is covered in section 11.2.5.2. Allergic responses in the oral cavity have multiple presentations, including erythema, erosion, edema, lichenoid reaction, itching, and/or gingival desquamation.

11.3.1   Oral allergy syndrome

Oral allergy syndrome (OAS) is a unique and rare condition that is characterized by itching, burning, and/or swelling of the lips, oral mucosa, tongue, and/or oropharynx in response to certain foods, in particular fruits, vegetables, and nuts. OAS is not a separate food allergy but rather represents a response to remnants of tree or wood pollen found in certain foods, and therefore only occurs in pollen-allergic patients. OAS is a type I hypersensitivity response, and consequently symptoms typically develop within a few minutes after eating the food. Patients presenting with symptoms suggestive of OAS should be referred to an allergist for further work-up. Diagnosis may consist of obtaining an accurate history of symptoms, maintenance of a food diary, skin/patch testing, and then food elimination followed by a food challenge.

11.3.2   Contact hypersensitivity

Contact hypersensitivity is a tissue response to potential allergens that come in direct contact with intraoral tissues, including food or food colorants, dental products (e.g., mouthwash), as well as dental materials found in restorations (amalgam), fixed crowns (gold/other metal), orthodontic wires/brackets (nickel/other metal), and prostheses (e.g., methylmethacrylate or polymethylmethacrylate used in the fabrication of temporary restorations, removable dentures, or orthodontic appliances; Figure 11.18). The clinical presentation varies, dependent upon the allergen and its direct contact with oral tissues. Food and dental products may cause a diffuse reaction, presenting as edema and erythema or

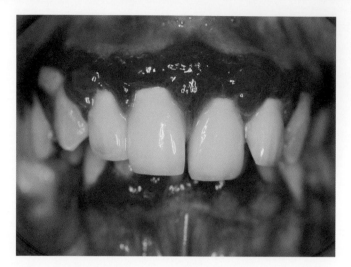

Figure 11.19 Plasma cell gingivitis on the maxillary arch of a young male. Note the brilliant erythematous appearance of the free and attached gingiva.

generalized mucosal sloughing. Allergy to acrylic often develops as erythema and edema of the mucosal surfaces in direct contact with acrylic and should be differentiated from an erythematous fungal infection (see chapter 7). Allergy to amalgam or metal materials typically presents as a lichenoid reaction on the mucosa adjacent to and in contact with the material (section 11.2.2).

Diagnosis of contact hypersensitivity begins with recognition of the offending allergen(s). The identification process for food or dental products as the potential allergen may be challenging, and ascertainment may require maintenance of a food and dental product intake diary. Removal of the potential food or dental product allergen should result in resolution of the lesion(s), thereby confirming the diagnosis. When a dental material is a suspected etiologic agent, there will be a temporal relationship between placement of the material and presentation of symptoms. Replacement with another material often results in clinical improvement of the affected tissue(s). Lichenoid mucosal changes may take longer to resolve and must be differentiated from other conditions with similar clinical characteristics. Therefore a biopsy of the involved area may contribute to diagnosis, as it will yield findings similar to that of lichenoid reactions (section 11.2.2). Allergy patch testing is generally not recommended.

11.3.3 *Plasma cell gingivitis*

Plasma cell gingivitis is a contact allergy characterized by intense gingival erythema and edema, discomfort, and bleeding with brushing (Figure 11.19). The affected area rarely spreads to the hard palate and may occur in edentulous areas with less intensity. The presumed etiology is an immune response to a known (e.g., toothpaste or prophylaxis paste) or unknown allergen. Since the condition is often persistent, diagnosis of plasma cell gingivitis requires a biopsy. Histologically, there is a dense population of plasma cells in the subepithelial gingival connective tissue, responsible for the erythematous and edematous lesion appearance and chronicity of the reaction. Patch testing is not recommended.

11.3.4 *Angioedema*

Angioedema is characterized by dysregulation of the complement system and allergic edema of soft tissues secondary to release of vast amounts of histamine (type I hypersensitivity), usually involving respiratory, gastrointestinal, and oral mucosa, including the lips. The clinical characteristics include extensive respiratory mucosal swelling that may cause an itching sensation and respiratory distress. The swelling may also involve other dermatologic surfaces, including the extremities, perioral area, and abdomen.

Angioedema is classified as hereditary or acquired. The hereditary type is associated with a quantitative or qualitative deficiency of C1-esterase inhibitor (C1-INH), and low levels of the enzyme are diagnostic for the condition. Acquired angioedema is primarily associated with use of ACE inhibitors, and discontinuation of the suspected medication leads to clinical resolution. Patch testing plays no role in the diagnosis of angioedema.

11.4   Suggested literature

Abraham C, Cho JH. Inflammatory bowel disease. N Engl J Med 2009;361:2066–2078.

Barnes J, Mayes MD. Epidemiology of systemic sclerosis: Incidence, prevalence, survival, risk factors, malignancy, and environmental triggers. Curr Opin Rheumatol 2012;24:165–170.

Chan LS. Ocular and oral mucous membrane pemphigoid (cicatricial pemphigoid). Clin Dermatol 2012 Jan;30:34–37.

Chi AC, Neville BW, Krayer JW, Gonsalves WC. Oral manifestations of systemic disease. Am Fam Physician 2010;82:1381–1388.

Daley TD, Armstrong JE. Oral manifestations of gastrointestinal diseases. Can J Gastroenterol 2007;21:241–244.

Iannuzzi MC, Rybicki BA, Teirstein AS. Sarcoidosis. N Engl J Med 2007;357:2153–2165.

Kamala KA, Ashok L, Annigeri RG. Herpes associated erythema multiforme. Contemp Clin Dent 2011;2:372–375.

Longhurst H, Cicardi M. Hereditary angio-oedema. Lancet 2012;379:474–481.

Sicherer SH, Leung DY. Advances in allergic skin disease, anaphylaxis, and hypersensitivity reactions to foods, drugs, and insects in 2011. J Allergy Clin Immunol 2012;129:76–85.

Suresh L, Neiders ME. Definitive and differential diagnosis of desquamative gingivitis through direct immunofluorescence studies. 2012 Jan 20:J Periodontol. [Epub ahead of print].

12 Orofacial Pain Conditions

12.0 INTRODUCTION

Pain is a subjective symptom defined by the International Association for the Study of Pain (IASP) as "an unpleasant sensory and emotional experience associated with actual or potential tissue damage, or described in terms of such damage." The diagnostic process to investigate a pain complaint may be straightforward, such as a toothache with clinically obvious caries and an acute pulpitis, or complex, which may involve physical, psychological, and social factors that can combine to create unique pain experiences. Orofacial pain is a presenting symptom of a broad spectrum of conditions affecting the orofacial complex (Table 12.1). There are numerous etiologies for pain symptoms, and, as with all pain conditions, the pain presentation can vary significantly. Some conditions are easily recognized and treated, while others are challenging to localize, and diagnosis and management may be difficult.

Orofacial pain complaints may involve teeth and their supporting structures or may be due to non-odontogenic causes. When assessing orofacial pain, the dental practitioner must first rule-out odontogenic etiology. Common odontogenic conditions such as dental caries and acute periodontal disease should be considered, as well as dentin hypersensitivity and cracked tooth syndrome. Further, inflammatory and/or infectious orofacial conditions often present with pain and may affect extraoral and/or intraoral hard and soft tissues. For example, lichen planus may be accompanied by tissue inflammation and ulceration, with common presenting symptoms being mucosal tissue pain or sensitivity. Another condition, osteomyelitis, is an acute or chronic bone infection that can occur in patients secondary to mandible fractures, odontogenic or soft tissue infection, or as a complication of a local or regional surgical procedure. Symptoms include deep pain and tenderness, swelling, erythema, and, in acute cases, fever. In general, extraoral and/or intraoral hard and soft tissue pathology typically presents with tissue changes or damage that corresponds to the pain complaint.

Other orofacial pain conditions are more complex, as they may represent pain referred to orofacial structures, pain that mimics toothache symptoms, or pain originating in orofacial structures that are not easy to visualize, such as muscular, vascular, and neural structures. These pain conditions will be addressed in this chapter. Diagnosis and management of

Risk Assessment and Oral Diagnostics in Clinical Dentistry, First Edition.
Dena J. Fischer, Nathaniel S. Treister and Andres Pinto.
© 2013 John Wiley & Sons, Inc. Published 2013 by John Wiley & Sons, Inc.

Table 12.1 Categories of non-odontogenic orofacial pain conditions.

System	Diagnosis	Signs and symptoms
Musculoskeletal	Temporomandibular disorders	Facial pain TMJ pain Pain in muscles of mastication
	Headache (muscular origin)	Bilateral pain in temporalis and/or pericranial muscles
Vascular	Giant cell arteritis (temporal arteritis, cranial arteritis)	Severe headache Tenderness in temporal region Visual disturbance Jaw claudication
	Migraine headache	Unilateral, severe facial pain May be associated with aura
	Trigeminal autonomic cephalgias (TACs)	*Cluster headache* unilateral, severe pain, rapid onset duration up to 3 hours assocated with periods of oxygen desaturation (e.g., sleep) autonomic changes: facial flushing, rhinorrhea, lacrimation, salivation, facial edema
		Chronic paroxysmal hemicrania unilateral, severe pain, rapid onset duration up to 45 minutes, multiple episodes per day may occur autonomic changes: sinus stuffiness, rhinorrhea, lacrimation, edema aborted with indomethacin
		Short-lasting unilateral neuralgiform headache with conjunctival injection and tearing/cranial autonomic features (SUNCT/SUNA) unilateral, severe pain, rapid onset duration a few seconds, high frequency of episodes orbital, supraorbital, temporal and frontal location autonomic changes: conjunctival injection and tearing
Neurologic	Trigeminal neuralgia Post-herpetic neuralgia	Severe, episodic, unilateral pain in nerve distribution History of herpes zoster Constant pain in nerve distribution corresponding to dermatome of herpes zoster presentation
	Chronic trigeminal neuropathy (post-traumatic neuropathic pain, atypical odontalgia)	Persistent pain, varies in intensity No odontogenic pathology

orofacial pain conditions can be challenging since the differential diagnosis is complex, multifactorial etiologic factors may contribute to the pain experience, and achievement of pain relief may be difficult. Complex orofacial pain conditions often require referral to pain specialists, and a timely and appropriate referral can minimize unnecessary dental procedures as well as improve quality of life and associated morbidity. An understanding of pain perception and pathways is necessary for the clinician to recognize these disorders when they present in the orofacial region.

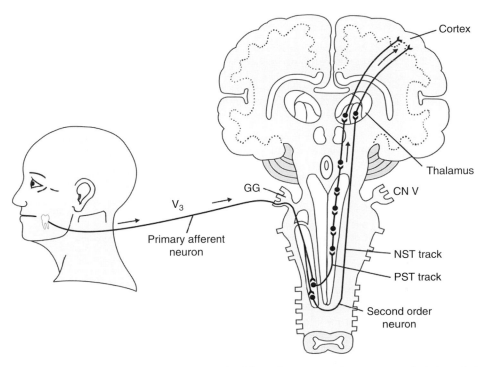

Figure 12.1   Afferent pain pathway. The impulse follows the primary afferent neuron of V3 through the gasserian ganglion (GG) into the subnucleus caudalis region of the trigeminal spinal tract, where it synapses with a second-order neuron and travels through the neospinothalamic tract (NST Tract) or paleospinothalamic tract (PST Tract) to the thalamus and cortex.
Reproduced with permission from Okeson JP. Bell's Orofacial Pains, 5th ed., Figure 3.2, page 54, Quintessence Publishing Co. Inc., Chicago.

12.1   Pain mechanisms

Pain is initiated through noxious stimulation of primary afferent neurons at the site of injury, and the signal is carried centrally through complex neurochemical processes (Figure 12.1). Orofacial pain is generated by sensory innervation supplied predominantly by the trigeminal nerve, though the facial (CNVII), glossopharyngeal (CNIX), vagus (CNX), and/or branches of the higher cervical nerves may also be involved. In the trigeminal nerve (CNV), most primary afferents converge in the trigeminal sensory ganglion, communicate with second-order neurons in the spinal nucleus of CNV, and transmit nociceptive input centrally to the thalamus and then the primary somatosensory cortex. Several primary afferents can converge to signal a single second-order neuron in the brain stem complex, resulting in pain referral and difficulties in pain localization. The autonomic nervous system also responds to painful stimulus through sympathetic and parasympathetic innervation, causing increased heart rate and other physiologic activities, including control over sweat glands, salivary flow, and pupil activity.

12.2   General classification of pain

Orofacial pain can be broadly classified as being either *nociceptive* or *neuropathic*. Nociceptive, or inflammatory, pain is transmitted by normal physiologic pathways in response to potentially tissue-damaging stimuli and typically ends when the underlying

Table 12.2 Characteristics of neuropathic pain.

Signs and Symptoms	Persistent pain caused by a lesion (including trauma) or disease of the somatosensory nervous system Diagnostic investigations reveal a sensory abnormality of affected nerve(s) and/or clinical history reveals trauma or disease that justifies diagnosis Clinical absence of pathology that may cause pain symptoms May affect central, peripheral, and/or autonomic nerves
Characteristics	Hyperalgesia: Increased response to a stimulus that is normally painful Allodynia: Pain due to a stimulus that does not normally provoke pain Paresthesia: Abnormal sensory sensation Dysesthesia: Abnormal and unpleasant sensation, whether spontaneous or evoked
Temporal Pattern	Episodic: Intense pain that varies in frequency and duration, associated with pain-free episodes Continuous: Constant pain that presents with varying intensities

tissue injury resolves. Pain may also be classified as *neuropathic*, in which pain is initiated or caused by a primary lesion, disease, or dysfunction in the nervous system, and nociceptor stimulation is not necessary (Table 12.2). While tissue and nerve injury may initiate processes that lead to pain, neuropathic pain persists once the initial injury heals due to damage and/or dysfunction in the pain-generating pathways. These alterations in pain processing at the peripheral and central levels produce characteristic symptoms such as *hyperalgesia* (an increased response to a stimulus that is normally painful), *allodynia* (pain due to a stimulus that does not normally provoke pain), *dysesthesia* (an unpleasant and abnormal sensation, whether spontaneous or evoked), and *paresthesia* (an abnormal sensation, whether spontaneous or evoked). Neuropathic pain can be an extremely debilitating form of pain that occurs when peripheral, autonomic, and/or central nerves are affected.

12.3 Pain assessment

Assessment of a pain patient involves numerous steps that begin with obtaining a pain history, followed by clinical assessment of the pain condition to include physical and functional assessment as well as possible imaging and laboratory studies. Finally, the behavioral contributions to the pain condition must be considered in all patients.

12.3.1 *Pain history*

Assessment of the patient with an orofacial pain complaint begins with a pain history and description of pain characteristics. This portion of the evaluation is critical in determining etiologic factors, orofacial structures that may be involved, and, ultimately, a definitive pain diagnosis. The pain history should involve a patient's description (self-report) of the intensity, persistence (continuous vs. episodic), and duration of overall pain, as well as duration of pain episodes and functional impact upon daily activities such as eating and sleeping. Pain intensity should be reported as "current," "worst," and "average" pain using a pain scale. For example, a categorical scale may classify the pain as none/mild/moderate/severe, or a numerical 0 to 10 scale may be utilized, with "0" representing no pain and "10" representing the worst pain one can imagine (Figure 12.2). The patient should also use adjectives

0   1   2   3   4   5   6   7   8   9   10

No pain   Worst possible pain

Figure 12.2   Numeric rating scale.

to describe his/her pain experience, such as "dull and achy" or "sharp and electrifying." Activities and/or treatments that increase the pain as well as those that decrease the pain experience, and to what degree the changes in pain occur, should be ascertained. Orofacial pain conditions that have been present for less than 3 months are generally categorized as acute conditions, while those that have persisted for at least 3 months are considered chronic pain conditions.

Potential etiologic factors contributing to the pain presentation should be elicited from the history, including recent dental procedures or a history of direct trauma to orofacial structures. The history should also recognize systemic conditions that may affect orofacial structures (e.g., arthritis conditions may affect the temporomandibular joints [TMJs]) and pain conditions that may present in orofacial structures (e.g., migraine headache). Parafunctional activities and recent stressful events should also be identified in the orofacial pain work-up.

12.3.2   Clinical pain assessment

The physical assessment involves thorough evaluation of the orofacial structures associated with the pain complaint and should begin with a patient pointing to the area(s) where s/he is experiencing the greatest source of pain. Extraorally, basic tests of balance and proprioception (standing without swaying, touching hand to nose) as well as sensory and motor function of cranial nerves should be assessed. Sensory evaluation involves determining if symptoms of hyperalgesia, allodynia, paresthesia, and/or anesthesia are present and should be performed when the pain history indicates altered sensory function, particularly along the three trigeminal nerve branches. For example, brushing a cotton-tipped applicator lightly along the CNV distribution may result in a sensation of light touch (normal), increased itchy or pain sensation (allodynia), decreased sensation (paresthesia), or no sensation (anesthesia). To assess for hyperalgesia, utilizing a "sharp" pointed instrument (e.g., the wooden end of a cotton-tipped applicator) along the nerve distribution may result in an increased pain response. Altered sensory function extending beyond the trigeminal nerve should be recorded during the examination and may warrant referral to a neurologist for further evaluation.

Next, the TMJs and surrounding structures should be assessed. During evaluation, the patient should report the pain presence and intensity using a ranking (e.g., none/mild/moderate/severe) or scale (e.g., 0-10 scale). The patient is instructed to open his/her mouth as wide as possible without pain, and the interincisal distance, known as the *range of mandibular movement* (ROM), is recorded (e.g., using a ruler or other measurement device). The patient is asked to close and then open as wide as possible even if there is pain and point to the area(s) that are most painful. A second measurement, the ROM with pain, is recorded. If the opening appears to be limited (less than 40 millimeters), the clinician should use the thumb and index finger to gently assist the patient to open farther. This is the *passive stretching* value and is helpful in distinguishing between limitations of ROM due to disc displacement without reduction (unable to assist the patient to open further; section 12.4.1) or other rare pathology (such as neoplasm) and muscular dysfunction (ability to increase ROM at least 5 millimeters with passive assistance). The open/close pattern of the mandible is recorded (straight, corrected deviation [S curve], uncorrected deviation). Next, the lateral poles of the TMJs, located anterior to the external meatus, are palpated for the presence of pain, indicating joint inflammation, and then opening and closing movements are performed to assess for the presence and timing (e.g., early or late in the masticatory cycle) of TMJ sounds (clicking, popping, and/or crepitus), pain, and palpable differences in joint form. Lateral and protrusive excursions are measured, and pain and/or joint sounds that occur during these movements should be recorded. Normal lateral and protrusive movements are at least 7 millimeters. Lastly, the bilateral extraoral muscles of mastication (temporalis, masseter) and cervical muscles (sternocleidomastoid, platysma, occipital, trapezius) are palpated using firm pressure and the patient is asked to report upon the presence and intensity of pain at each site of muscle palpation and whether or not palpation produces pain beyond the site being evaluated (pain referral).

Intraoral examination begins with palpation of bilateral intraoral muscles of mastication (masseter, lateral pterygoid) and recording the presence and intensity of pain. Changes in occlusion manifesting as a unilateral or bilateral open bite should be recorded, as they may indicate joint remodeling or destruction and can be slowly progressive or rapid in development. If indicated by the history of the pain complaint, evaluation of odontogenic structures may include palpation, percussion, thermal sensitivity testing, periodontal probing, and/or factors related to occlusion. Finally, if sensory alterations of the intraoral CNV maxillary and/or mandibular nerve branches are suspected from the pain history, evaluation of hyperalgesia, allodynia, paresthesia, and/or anesthesia should be performed.

12.3.3   *Diagnostic imaging*

Radiographs are not required in all circumstances of orofacial pain. The decision regarding use of imaging should be based upon whether or not radiographic findings may contribute to the diagnosis and/or may affect clinical care. With intraoral pain complaints, bitewing and periapical radiographs may be considered to rule-out odontogenic conditions, and in some cases occlusal films may be warranted; for example, to assess for salivary gland obstruction or alveolar bone expansion. Imaging of extraoral structures may be indicated if pain is chronic, progressive, or non-responsive to conservative treatment. For example, if occlusal changes are noted or pain localized to the TMJ is noted during examination, TMJ images may illustrate degenerative (arthritic) changes. Panoramic films provide basic information about the TMJs but are of limited diagnostic value since they are two-dimensional images of three-dimensional structures, and visualization may be further obstructed by superimposition of multiple structures. Computed tomography (CT) and cone beam CT may be used to assess the TMJs and other orofacial hard tissues. If alterations of soft tissue structures are suspected in the pain etiology, such as TMJ disc disorders, neoplastic disease or neurologic change, magnetic resonance imaging (MRI) can provide detailed imaging of the articular disc and other soft tissue structures (Figures 12.3 and 12.4). MRIs of the TMJs are typically performed in open and closed jaw positions to identify the articular disc location during jaw movement, and inflammatory changes can be visualized with T2-weighted images.

12.3.4   *Other diagnostic modalities*

In some circumstances, diagnostic nerve blocks may be useful when trying to distinguish between the site of the pain (the location of the pain presentation) and the source of the pain (the orofacial structures causing the pain). For example, in the case of pain presenting

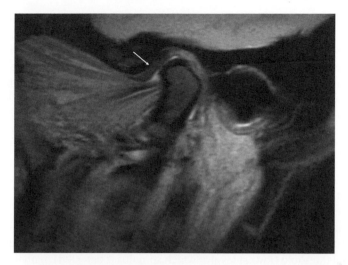

Figure 12.3 T1-weighted MRI of the left temporomandibular joint. The jaw is closed, as indicated by the position of the condyle relative to the articular eminence. The articular disk, which is radiolucent (arrow), is in a normal position relative to the condyle.

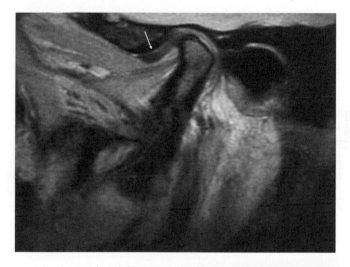

Figure 12.4 T1-weighted MRI of the left temporomandibular joint. The jaw is in a closed position. The articular disk, which is radiolucent (arrow), is anteriorly displaced relative to the condyle.

in the masseter muscle when the source is expected to be odontogenic (e.g., pulp, periodontium), anesthesia of odontogenic structure eliminates the symptom of facial pain. Diagnostic blocks may also be beneficial in determining which nerve branch(es) are involved in the pain or altered sensory distribution when neuropathic pain is suspected. If nerve dysfunction is located in the peripheral branches of the nerve only, anesthesia to the affected area will usually extinguish the pain or altered sensation. However, if the nerve dysfunction is more centrally located, anesthesia will not affect the pain presentation. Diagnostic nerve block results can be equivocal with centrally mediated pain conditions (e.g., trigeminal neuralgia, post-herpetic neuralgia; section 12.4.2) and may not contribute to a diagnosis.

Laboratory tests for autoimmune disease may be considered if systemic autoimmune arthritic conditions (e.g., rheumatoid arthritis, psoriatic arthritis, systemic lupus erythematosus) are suspected in the etiology of temporomandibular disorders (TMDs), particularly when the clinical presentation involves bilateral joint pain and swelling (see chapter 11). If tests are positive or if systemic disease is suspected, the patient should be referred to a physician for further evaluation.

An orofacial pain condition termed giant cell arteritis (GCA) is a chronic inflammatory disorder that often affects the temporal artery (section 12.4.3.2). The gold standard diagnostic test for GCA is a temporal artery biopsy, and a positive specimen will demonstrate a chronic inflammatory infiltrate with destruction of the internal elastic lamina. In addition, confirmatory laboratory tests include an elevated erythrocyte sedimentation rate (ESR) and C-reactive protein (CRP).

Quantitative sensory testing (QST) is a set of sensory tests (thermal, mechanical/tactile, electrical) utilized for the assessment of sensory abnormalities. QST modalities selectively activate different sensory nerve fibers, and upon stimulation, sensation is evaluated/assessed by the detection threshold (lowest level at which stimulus is detected), pain threshold (lowest level at which pain is detected), and pain tolerance (highest level at which pain is tolerated). While QST may be employed in clinical settings, its use for orofacial pain assessment is typically limited to research.

12.3.5   Behavioral aspects of pain

It is well recognized that psychological and social factors can contribute to augmentation or diminishment of a patient's pain experience and reporting. These behavioral factors have a greater impact with chronic pain conditions, where psychosocial contributors such as depression, anxiety, and somatization (the conversion of anxiety into physical symptoms) may significantly contribute to the pain experience. Studies of chronic pain have demonstrated that high scores of depression or somatization are strong predictors of pain severity and persistence. Further, in the presence of chronic pain conditions, patients may have a diminished ability to cope with their pain. Consequently, when assessing patients with chronic orofacial pain conditions, it is critical to consider psychosocial factors in addition to the physical pain assessment. A chronic pain patient may warrant referral to a pain specialist to manage the pain condition and/or a mental health specialist to assess levels of depression, anxiety, and somatization as well as the patient's ability to cope with the pain condition.

The degree of pain dysfunction is a strong indicator of pain chronicity and may be evaluated in the dental office using behavioral questionnaires commonly utilized in behavioral and pain research. The Axis II component of the *Research Diagnostic Criteria (RDC) for Temporomandibular Disorders* is a questionnaire that assesses several important psychosocial contributors to pain. Two important components of the Axis II are the *Characteristic Pain Intensity* (CPI), which measures the overall pain intensity over time, and *Pain Disability*, which measures the impact of the pain on the patient's ability to engage in normal daily activities, such as employment, housework and family and social duties. The CPI and Pain Disability scales are combined to determine the *Graded Chronic Pain* (GCP) score, which indicates the level of pain dysfunction (Figure 12.5). Patients with GCP levels of I or II are less likely to develop chronic pain, and seem to respond more favorably to conservative treatments, while patients with GCP levels of III or IV are more likely to experience chronic and persistent pain.

1. How would you rate your facial pain on a 0 to 10 scale at the present time, that is right now, where 0 is "no pain" and 10 is "pain as bad as could be"?

0   1   2   3   4   5   6   7   8   9   10
No pain   Pain as bad as could be

2. In the past six months, how intense was your worst pain rated on a 0 to 10 scale where 0 is "no pain" and 10 is "pain as bad as could be"?

0   1   2   3   4   5   6   7   8   9   10
No pain   Pain as bad as could be

3. In the past six months, on the average, how intense was your pain rated on a 0 to 10 scale where 0 is "no pain" and 10 is "pain as bad as could be" [That is, your usual pain at times you were experiencing pain]?

0   1   2   3   4   5   6   7   8   9   10
No pain   Pain as bad as could be

4. In the past six months, how much has facial pain interfered with your daily activities rated on a 0 to 10 scale where 0 is "no interference" and 10 is "unable to carry on any activities"?

0   1   2   3   4   5   6   7   8   9   10
No interference   Unable to carry on any activities

5. In the past six months, how much has facial pain changed your ability to take part in recreational, social and family activities where 0 is "no change" and 10 is "extreme change"?

0   1   2   3   4   5   6   7   8   9   10
No change   Extreme change

6. In the past six months, how much has facial pain changed your ability to work (including housework) where 0 is "no change" and 10 is "extreme change"?

0   1   2   3   4   5   6   7   8   9   10
No change   Extreme change

7. About how many days in the last six months have you been kept from your usual activities (work, school, or housework) because of facial pain?

CHARACTERISTIC PAIN INTENSITY (CPI)

CPI: [Q1] + [Q2] + [Q3] = _____ divided by 3 = _____ × 10 = CPI Score

PAIN DISABILITY

Disability Days = [Q7]

0–6 days = 0 Disability Points
7–14 days = 1 Disability Point
15–30 days = 2 Disability Points
31+ days = 3 Disability Points

Disability Score: [Q4] + [Q5] + [Q6] = _____ divided by 3 = _____ × 10 = Disability Score

Disability Score of 0–29 = 0 Disability Points
Disability Score of 30–49 = 1 Disability Point
Disability Score of 50–69 = 2 Disability Points
Disability Score of 70+ = 3 Disability Points

Total Disability Points = (points for Disability Days) + (points for Disability Score)

CHRONIC PAIN GRADE (CPG) CLASSIFICATION

CPG classification		Defining characteristics
Low disability	Grade I, Low Intensity	CPI < 50, and < 3 Disability Points
	Grade II, High Intensity	CPI ≥ 50, and < 3 Disability Points
High disability	Grade III, Moderately Limiting	3–4 Disability Points, regardless of CPI
	Grade IV, Severely Limiting	5–6 Disability Points, regardless of CPI

Figure 12.5 Graded Chronic Pain Scale and Assessment. Reference: von Korff M, Ormal J, Dworkin SF. Grading the severity of chronic pain. Pain 1992;15:133–149.

Table 12.3 Diagnostic categories of temporomandibular disorders.

Diagnostic category	Diagnosis	Signs and symptoms
Articular bone (joint)	Arthralgia (capsulitis)	Pain upon palpation of TMJ Self-reports of joint pain
	Arthritis (osteoarthritis or degenerative joint disease)	Arthralgia Crepitus in TMJ and/or osseous changes visible on radiographic imaging
	Arthrosis	No arthralgia Crepitus in TMJ and/or osseous changes visible on radiographic imaging
Muscular	Myofascial pain	Pain upon palpation of muscles of mastication
	Myofascial pain with limited opening	Pain upon palpation of muscles of mastication Limited opening (< 35 mm) and ability to increase ROM (≥ 5 mm) with passive assistance
	Myositis	Constant, acute pain in a localized muscle area Limited ROM due to acute pain and swelling
Articular disc (internal derangement)	Disc displacement with reduction	Click/pop in TMJ upon opening/closing No limited ROM due to disc condition
	Disc displacement without reduction with limited opening (acute disc displacement)	Limited opening (< 35 mm) Inability to increase ROM with passive assistance and decrease in contralateral excursive movement, OR Uncorrected deviation to ipsilateral side on opening
	Disc displacement without reduction (chronic disc displacement)	History of limitation in opening, no limited opening currently Minimal to no limitation in contralateral excursive movement
	Spontaneous displacement	Mouth in wide-open position Inability to close

12.4 Classification and diagnosis of pain conditions

12.4.1 *Temporomandibular disorders*

Temporomandibular disorders are a collection of nociceptive pain disorders involving the soft tissue structures within the joint, muscles of mastication, and/or articular bones of the TMJ (Table 12.3). TMD affects almost two times as many females as males, and the most prevalent age group is individuals between the ages of 20 and 40 years. In older adults with TMD complaints, *osteoarthritis*, or *degenerative joint disease*, is the most common etiology.

There are a number of classification systems for TMD, and in general these systems establish a diagnosis of TMD categorized into subtypes of articular disc, muscular, and/or joint (articular bone) disorders. The RDC for TMD, currently being revised and termed

Diagnostic Criteria for TMD is one classification system that was developed for research purposes but has been used in clinical arenas and has been translated into numerous languages. Another classification system published by the American Academy of Orofacial Pain attempts to define the diagnostic terms and provides clinical criteria to a comprehensive list of TMD diagnoses.

Disc disorders may also be termed *internal derangements* of the TMJ and are characterized by an abnormal relationship between the articular disc, condyle, and articular eminence, resulting from elongation or sometimes tearing of the ligaments attached to the disc. A diagnosis of *TMJ disc displacement with reduction* is made when a click or popping sound emanates from the TMJ with opening and closing movements. There may be a limitation in jaw opening if a muscle disorder is also present, but there is no limitation of opening due to the disc condition. The click/pop detected with jaw closing is often softer than the opening noise and may or may not be heard. A diagnosis of *TMJ disc displacement without reduction with limited opening* is characterized by a limited ROM (less than about 35 millimeters) and (a) an inability to increase the ROM (less than 5 millimeters) with passive assistance plus a decrease in contralateral excursive movement (less than 7 millimeters), and/or (b) an uncorrected deviation to the ipsilateral side on opening. This condition may be detected in a patient who has a history of TMJ disc displacement with reduction, whose symptoms progress to intermittent locking episodes, followed by a sudden restriction in mandibular opening. A diagnosis of *TMJ disc displacement without reduction (chronic disc displacement)* is made when the patient has a long (at least 2- to 3-month) history of limitation in opening but has recovered to a current ROM that is not limited (greater than 35 millimeters) plus minimal to no limitation in contralateral excursive movement. This diagnosis may be confirmed with MRI imaging of the TMJs (Figure 12.4) and is signified by the articular disc deforming after having been chronically displaced and the repositioning of the retrodiscal tissues (posterior attachment) to the location between the condyle and articular eminence, where they become a fibrous connective tissue *"pseudodisc."* A *spontaneous displacement*, also referred to as an *"open lock,"* can occur when the condyle is translated to its anterior limit and the disc is displaced anterior or posterior to the condyle. This diagnosis is made when the mouth is in a wide-open position with inability to close.

For the muscular disorders, the most common diagnosis is *myofascial pain* (pain in muscles and surrounding fascial tissue), characterized by pain upon palpation of the muscles of mastication. Myofascial pain may be associated with limited jaw opening due to inflammation and protective guarding, but the ROM can increase at least 5 millimeters with passive stretching. *Myositis* is defined as inflammation and swelling of a muscle and is signified by constant, acute pain in a localized muscle area, resulting in a limited range of motion due to acute pain and swelling.

Inflammation in the synovial fluid of the joint space may occur secondary to disc and/or articular bone disorders. Osteoarthritis (degenerative joint disease) is a localized condition in which the articular cartilage degrades and fibroses, leading to sclerosis as well as subchondral cyst and osteophyte formation of the underlying articular bone (Figure 12.6). These bony changes typically undergo remodeling and may be asymptomatic unless accompanied by secondary inflammation of the synovial membrane. The articular bone diagnoses are *arthralgia (capsulitis)*, *arthritis*, and *arthrosis*. Arthralgia, also sometimes referred to as "capsulitis," is characterized by pain in one or both of the TMJs during palpation plus self-reports of joint pain. Arthritis is defined as arthralgia plus crepitus in the TMJ and/or osseous changes (narrowing of the joint space, flattening of the articular surfaces, osteophyte or subchondral cyst formation, anterior lipping of the condyle) visible on radiographic imaging

(a)   (b)

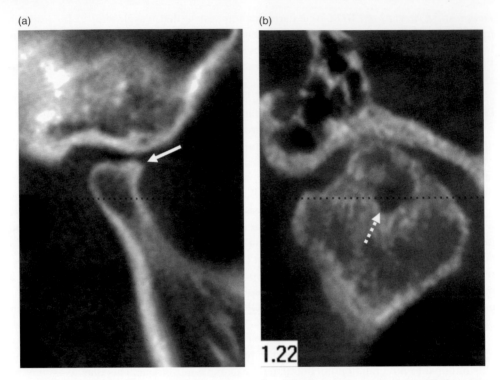

Figure 12.6 Cone beam computed tomography (CBCT) of the temporomandibular joints. (a) Degenerative joint changes of the right TMJ with flattening of the glenoid fossa, osteophytic growth at the anterior margin of the head of the condyle, and anterior lipping of the condyle (solid arrow); (b) the right TMJ shows degenerative joint changes signified by widening of the glenoid fossa, sclerosis of the roof of the glenoid fossa, and osteophyte formation at the anterior margin of the condylar head. The well-circumscribed, homogeneous radiolucency is a subchondral bone "cyst" (broken arrow) that corresponds to an area of osseous degeneration that typically contains fibrous and/or granulation tissue. Figures courtesy of Dr. Richard Monahan, University of Illinois at Chicago.

(Figure 12.6). Arthrosis is defined as crepitus in the TMJ and/or osseous changes present with radiographic imaging with the absence of arthralgia.

Management of TMDs initially consists of conservative treatment to include patient education, reversal of habitual jaw activities (clenching, leaning on jaw), eliminating aggravating factors, physical therapy (cold and moist heat therapy, passive jaw-stretching activities), short-term pharmacotherapy (anti-inflammatory and/or muscle relaxation medication), and the use of an intraoral appliance. Further intervention such as behavioral/relaxation techniques, trigger-point injections, intense physical therapy, and/or addressing psychosocial contributors may be warranted, and appropriate referral should be considered.

12.4.2 Neuropathic pain

Neuropathic pain conditions can be classified into two categories based upon the temporal pattern of the pain: *episodic* and *continuous* (Table 12.2). Episodic pain is characterized by sudden and brief but intense electric-like pain that may be spontaneous or provoked by mechanical stimuli or movement and is associated with pain-free episodes. Continuous neuropathic pain presents with constant, unremitting pain, often described as dull, aching,

---

Alert Box   12.1   Signs of elevated suspicion for a craniofacial tumor or lesion.

Unilateral motor loss/dysfunction
Visual disturbances
Unilateral symptoms mimicking trigeminal neuralgia in younger patients (<50 years old)

---

throbbing, or burning, and may have periods of greater or lesser intensity. The diagnosis of a neuropathic pain condition is typically based on the positive history for pain descriptors that indicate severe pain intensity and sensory abnormalities. Further, the physical examination and imaging studies illustrate an absence of obvious pain etiology, and clinical findings of hyperesthesia, allodynia, and/or paresthesia are present. Patients with persistent pain often seek consultation from many clinicians and undergo multiple unnecessary procedures before receiving a correct diagnosis and appropriate treatment.

12.4.2.1   *Episodic neuropathic pain*
Trigeminal neuralgia (TN) is an episodic neuropathic pain syndrome, described as a sharp, electrifying, shooting, stabbing, severe pain that follows one or more branches of CNV. The pain episode may occur spontaneously or may be triggered by light touch to a localized intra- or extraoral site, facial or tongue movement, or performing oral hygiene. The frequency and duration are variable, from an episode every few months to multiple episodes daily, lasting a few seconds to a few minutes. Following a painful attack, there is a refractory period, during which provocation of the trigger zone will not precipitate pain. The pain is almost always unilateral and if bilateral, an abnormality such as a central tumor or multiple sclerosis must be considered (Alert Box 12.1). Prior to diagnosing a patient with TN, appropriate referral is necessary, and an MRI of the head and brain may be warranted to rule-out underlying pathology.

12.4.2.2   *Continuous neuropathic pain*
Continuous neuropathic pain that persists for at least 3 months may be further classified into *neuritis* and *deafferentation* conditions. *Neuritis* is an inflammatory condition of the peripheral distribution of the nerve due to trauma, chemical, viral, or infectious causes, while *deafferentation* indicates trauma (crushing or cutting) of a peripheral nerve.

A prime example of *neuritis* is the persistent pain that can develop following herpes zoster infection, known as post-herpetic neuralgia (PHN). This neuropathic pain syndrome exhibits features of hyperalgesia and allodynia and is described as constant, mild to severe, and burning, deep aching, tingling, itching, and/or stabbing pain. The risk for PHN increases with age, and prevention of herpes zoster is available with the varicella zoster vaccine. For patients who develop herpes zoster, use of antiviral and anti-inflammatory drugs early in the course of disease may reduce the risk of PHN.

A number of terms have been used to describe *deafferentation* trigeminal neuropathies associated with trauma, such as chronic trigeminal neuropathy, post-traumatic neuropathic pain, atypical odontalgia, and non-odontogenic toothache. The traumatic event may be pulp extirpation, tooth extraction, or a routine dental procedure (e.g., scaling and root planing) that inadvertently causes trauma to a peripheral nerve. A chronic trigeminal neuropathy typically presents as prolonged periods of constant dull, deep, aching pain with occasional spontaneous sharp pain in a tooth or tooth region, in the absence of odontogenic etiology observed clinically or radiographically. It usually persists for months or years, being continuous and persistent but varying in intensity. Patients may have difficulty localizing the pain, and the location may change. There is usually a variable response to local anesthetic blocks. To further complicate diagnosis, the tooth or tooth region may exhibit hyperalgesia demonstrated by a positive response to percussion, sensitivity to cold, or pain associated with chewing; therefore, odontogenic etiologies such as a fractured tooth or failed root canal therapy should be ruled-out. It is not uncommon for patients to undergo multiple treatments including endodontic procedures and tooth extractions in a continued attempt to relieve the pain. As treatment is directed toward the "symptomatic" tooth, the symptoms often spread or move to adjacent teeth, and the pain quality (characteristics used to describe the pain) may change. Once a diagnosis is established, further dental procedures that could aggravate the pain must be avoided.

Management of neuropathic pain conditions consists of anticonvulsant medications, tricyclic antidepressants, and/or opioids. Topical medications such as capsaicin creams may provide some relief. Combination therapy and consultation with a pain management specialist are often required. For TN, neurosurgical procedures may be considered if a patient is not responsive to pharmacotherapeutic intervention.

12.4.3   Other pain conditions

12.4.3.1   Burning mouth syndrome

Burning mouth syndrome (BMS) is a chronic pain syndrome that is defined by the IASP as burning pain in the tongue or other oral mucous membranes lasting at least 4–6 months, with normal clinical and laboratory findings. BMS primarily affects females in the fifth to seventh decade, with a female-to-male ratio of about 7:1. The burning sensation is typically bilateral, moderate in severity, and may be constant, progressively increasing throughout the day, or intermittent. Unilateral symptoms require careful investigation to rule-out underlying disease (Alert Box 12.1). Remission of burning usually occurs with sleeping and may be less severe or absent when eating, chewing gum, or using an oral lozenge. Associated symptoms may include xerostomia without obvious hyposalivation, paresthesias, and altered taste (e.g., bitter, metallic). Over half the patients with BMS may experience a spontaneous onset of symptoms, while about 25% attribute onset to an identifiable triggering factor, suggesting the possibility of peripheral and/or central neurologic alterations preceding burning.

Diagnosis of BMS is made by obtaining a careful history and excluding possible causes, including local pathology of the mucosal tissues, salivary hypofunction, and medication side effects. If the review of systems suggests an underlying systemic disease, referring to a physician is warranted to rule-out systemic conditions that may cause oral burning, such as diabetes mellitus, anemia, nutritional deficiencies, hormonal disturbances, and psychiatric disorders. Treatment options such as tricyclic antidepressants, anticonvulsants, and topical and systemic clonazepam (a benzodiazepine derivative) have demonstrated efficacy in clinical trials.

12.4.3.2   Giant cell arteritis

Giant cell arteritis, also known as *cranial arteritis* or *temporal arteritis*, is a chronic inflammatory disorder involving large and medium-sized vessels with a tendency to affect the extracranial branches of the carotid artery, most commonly the temporal artery. Chronic inflammatory infiltrates affect the inner walls of arteries with classic histopathologic findings including granulomatous inflammation and multinucleated giant cells. Clinically, visual disturbances such as blurred vision, diplopia, and eye pain are often early manifestations of the disease. Other symptoms include fever, malaise, and weight loss, as well as temporal or occipital headache, tenderness in the temporal region, and jaw claudication (fatigue or pain on function).

Vestibular dysfunction and/or hearing impairment may also occur. Palpation of the involved superficial temporal arteries typically demonstrates a tender and thickened pulsating vessel. This condition usually develops in adults over 50 years old.

Diagnostic findings include an elevated ESR above 50 millimeters/hour (normal is 20 mm/hr or less) and elevated CRP greater than 40 milligrams/liter (normal is less than 10 mg/L). Temporal artery biopsy (performed by a vascular surgeon or other qualified medical professional) remains the gold standard to confirm the diagnosis of GCA, demonstrating a chronic inflammatory infiltrate with destruction of the internal elastic lamina. Long-term and severe complications of GCA include vision loss, stroke, and aortic aneurysm as a result of chronic vasculitis. Treatment with systemic corticosteroids must be initiated promptly to reduce the risk of blindness and stroke.

12.4.3.3   *Atypical facial pain*

Atypical facial pain (AFP) is described as a persistent pain involving the head and/or face that does not have the characteristics of other orofacial pain conditions. The International Headache Society defines AFP as "facial pain not fulfilling other criteria." Use of the term is controversial since true diagnostic criteria do not exist, and its use in classification systems is often reserved for individuals with facial pain that does not fall into other diagnostic categories.

The diagnosis of AFP is complex because there are so many possible causes of chronic facial pain. The diagnostic process must include a comprehensive assessment to rule-out other conditions, and if a specific cause for the pain is not identified, the diagnosis of AFP can be considered and tentatively applied or used as the working diagnosis.

12.4.3.4   *Sympathetically maintained pain*

Sympathetically maintained pain (SMP), also known as *complex regional pain syndrome*, is a complex, rare pain condition that is preceded by significant injury (e.g., motor vehicle accident, work-related injury) and has features of neuropathic pain that extends beyond the affected area. The disorder may be accompanied by autonomic changes in the affected region, such as flushing, altered local skin temperature, excessive sweating, and motor dysfunction; however, autonomic dysfunction is not required for a diagnosis of SMP. Allodynia, hyperalgesia, and spontaneous pain are common symptoms, and movement exacerbates the pain. Diagnosis of SMP involves elimination of symptoms when sympathetic activity to the affected region is blocked. Thus, the diagnostic test for SMP requires blockade of the sympathetic nervous system by either (a) local anesthetic blockage of the stellate ganglion, performed by an anesthesiologist, or (b) intravenous administration of phentolamine, an alpha-adrenergic antagonist. Management of this complex condition requires a multidisciplinary approach to chronic pain.

12.4.3.5   *Headache*

Headache conditions may have features that overlap with orofacial disorders or dental pathology. Consequently, it is important for the dental provider to differentiate signs and symptoms of headache disorders from dental disease and TMD. Headache may be muscular and/or vascular in origin and may contain characteristics of both types of pain, particularly in chronic headache sufferers.

The most common headache disorders include tension-type and migraine headache (Table 12.1). Tension-type headache is the most common type of headache and is muscular in origin, typically presenting as bilateral, steady, mild-to-moderate discomfort that is not severe or disabling. These headaches vary in duration, from 30 minutes to 7 days, and may be associated with pericranial muscular tenderness upon manual palpation. Migraine headache is the most common type of vascular headache and occasionally can cause pain in the face, jaws, or even odontogenic structures. Migraines are characterized by unilateral, throbbing or pulsating, moderate-to-severe pain that may be associated with an aura (prodrome) phase. They may involve the presence of nausea, photophobia, phonophobia, and/or pain worsening with activity. A typical migraine episode will last from 4 to 72 hours and often is relieved by sleep, a feature that distinguishes migraine headache from dental disease.

Another group of vascular headache disorders, called the trigeminal autonomic cephalgias (TACs), are far less frequently encountered headaches that are often associated with autonomic changes and may be confused with odontogenic and other orofacial pain conditions. TACs are unilateral, severely painful headaches that occur with rapid onset and are classified by the duration of headache symptoms. Cluster headache is a severely painful, unilateral headache condition, with episodes lasting a few minutes up to 3 hours. Attacks occur with a rapid onset and are more frequent during periods of oxygen desaturation, such as during sleep. Autonomic changes including facial flushing, rhinorrhea, lacrimation, salivation, and facial edema may occur. During episodes, structures in the region of the headache are often hypersensitive, and if dental structures are involved, pain can often mimic odontogenic symptoms. Chronic paroxysmal hemicrania is another TAC that presents with severe, unilateral pain and rapid onset. Pain episodes often last a few minutes up to 45 minutes, and multiple episodes per day may occur. The orbital, supraorbital, and temporal areas may be involved, and these headaches are typically aborted with indomethacin (a nonsteroidal anti-inflammatory drug). Autonomic changes include sinus stuffiness, rhinorrhea, lacrimation, and edema of the involved region. A third TAC is the short-lasting unilateral neuralgiform headache with conjunctival injection and tearing/cranial autonomic features (SUNCT/SUNA). These headaches have the shortest duration of the TACs, typically lasting a few seconds but with high frequency, from one per day to more than sixty per hour. The SUNCT/SUNA disorders are characterized by unilateral, severe pain in the orbital, supraorbital, temporal and frontal areas with autonomic features, such as conjunctival injection and tearing. Patients suffering with headache symptoms or suspected of having a headache disorder should be referred to a neurologist for evaluation and management.

12.5   Selected literature

Balasubramaniam R, Klasser GD, Delcanho R. Trigeminal autonomic cephalgias. JADA 2008;139(12): 1616–1624.

Clark GT. Persistent orodental pain, atypical odontalgia, and phantom tooth pain: When are they neuropathic disorders? J Calif Dent Assoc 2006;34(8):599–609.

Clark GT, Seligman DA, Solberg WK, Pullinger AG. Guidelines for the examination and diagnosis of temporomandibular disorders. J Craniomandib Disord 1989;3:7–14.

Dworkin S, LeResche L. Research diagnostic criteria for temporomandibular disorders: Review, criteria, examinations, and specifications, critique. J Craniomandib Disord 1992;6:301–335.

Eberhardt RT, Dhadly M. Giant cell arteritis: Diagnosis, management, and cardiovascular implications. Cardiol Rev 2007;15(2):55–61.

International RDC-TMD Consortium website, www.rdc-tmdinternational.org

Jung BF, Johnson RW, Griffin DR, Dworkin RH. Risk factors for postherpetic neuralgia in patients with herpes zoster. Neurology 2004;62(9):1545–1551.

Kurita K, Westesson PL, Yuasa H, et al. Natural course of untreated symptomatic temporomandibular joint disc displacement without reduction. J Dent Res 1998;77:361–365.

Merskey H, Bogduk N, eds. Classification of Chronic Pain, Task Force on Taxonomy, International Association for the Study of Pain, 2nd ed. Seattle: IASP Press, 1994.

National Institutes of Health Technology Assessment Conference on Management of Temporomandibular Disorders. Oral Surg Oral Med Oral Pathol Oral Radiol Endod 1997;83:49–183.

Okeson J, ed. Orofacial Pain: Guidelines for Assessment, Diagnosis, and Management. Chicago: Quintessence, 1996. [Clinical findings accompanying the diagnosis in AAOP publication on orofacial pain guidelines].

Ram S, Teruel A, Kumar SK, Clark G. Clinical characteristics and diagnosis of atypical odontalgia: Implications for dentists. JADA 2009;140(2):223–228.

Schiffman E, Anderson G, Fricton J. Diagnostic criteria for intra-articular TM disorders. Community Dent Oral Epidemiol 1989;17:252–257.

Schiffman EL, Ohrbach R, Truelove EL, et al. The Research Diagnostic Criteria for Temporomandibular Disorders. V: Methods used to establish and validate revised axis I diagnostic algorithms. J Orofac Pain 2010;24:63–78.

Appendix

Top 10 List of Non-odontogenic Oral Conditions

Oral Condition	Clinical Presentation	Signs and Symptoms	Clinical Implications
Fibroma	Firm, raised, pink nodule May appear white if traumatized	Usually asymptomatic May be painful if traumatized	Excision if bothersome
Hemangioma	Onset in childhood Raised nodules or flat lesions that appear red, blue, and/or purple in color Diascopy (palpation using pressure) may produce blanching	Typically asymptomatic Often involute with time without intervention May present bruit on palpation	Diagnosis typically well established since childhood Intraoral involvement may be associated with tissue deformities
Herpes Simplex Virus (HSV)	Primary gingivostomatitis: multiple lip and oral ulcerations Recurrent herpes labialis: coalescing vesicles on lip, crust with healing Recurrent intraoral herpes: shallow, irregular clusters of surface erosions that coalesce, occur on keratinized tissue	Primary gingivostomatitis: fever, lymphadenopathy Recurrent herpes: tingling (prodrome phase) Primary and recurrent intraoral lesions associated with severe pain	Active virus can be transferred from one individual to another or from one site to another on the same individual Management with topical and/or systemic antiviral medications Prophylactic management may be warranted on medically complex
Leukoplakia	White or mixed red/white in appearance Patch or plaque that cannot be scraped off Over time, a raised mass, ulceration, and/or induration may develop	May be asymptomatic May present with pain or discomfort	Considered a potentially malignant condition Requires biopsy for diagnosis Requires close follow-up and monitoring

(Continued)

Risk Assessment and Oral Diagnostics in Clinical Dentistry, First Edition.
Dena J. Fischer, Nathaniel S. Treister and Andres Pinto.
© 2013 John Wiley & Sons, Inc. Published 2013 by John Wiley & Sons, Inc.

(Cont'd)

Oral Condition	Clinical Presentation	Signs and Symptoms	Clinical Implications
Lichen Planus	Hyperkeratotic white soft tissue reticulations (Wickham striae) Erythema and ulcerations or tissue erosion, typically seen in association with reticular changes Buccal mucosa and tongue most common, but all oral tissues can be affected	Pain, usually with function Sensitivity when eating acidic and/or spicy foods Sensation of tightness of the oral cavity with wide opening	Management with topical and/or systemic steroids; some cases may require systemic immunomodulatory agents Requires long-term monitoring for potentially malignant changes
Mucocele (Mucous Extravasation Phenomenon)	Soft, fluctuant (fluid-filled) raised mass Translucent or faintly blue in color Lower lip most common site, but may occur at any site where minor salivary glands are located	Usually asymptomatic	Requires surgical excision
Oral Candidiasis	Raised multiple patchy white plaques that can generally be scraped away (pseudomembraneous form) Erythematous tissue, often seen on the palate under a denture (erythematous/atrophic form) Erythema and cracking of the corners of the mouth (angular cheilitis)	Burning, sensitivity, altered taste Cracking and sensitivity at corners of mouth	Management with antifungal medications Prophylactic management may be warranted in medically complex patients
Recurrent Aphthous Ulcerations	Small ovoid ulcers surrounded by erythematous halo Limited to non-keratinized tissue	Pain, especially with function	May be associated with stress, certain foods, heredity, or systemic conditions such as inflammatory bowel disease or Behcet syndrome If frequent recurrences, may be managed with topical steroids and/or systemic immodulatory agents
Salivary Hypofunction	Dry oral tissues Thick saliva, sometimes foamy or ropey	Difficulty eating hard/dry foods Difficulty swallowing Difficulty speaking Oral discomfort	Management with topical or systemic sialogogues Increased risk of secondary caries and/or fungal infection

(Continued)

(Cont'd)

Oral Condition	Clinical Presentation	Signs and Symptoms	Clinical Implications
Temporomandibular Disorders	Pain upon palpation of temporomandibular joint(s) and/or muscles of mastication May or may not present with limited opening Joint sounds (pop/click/crepitus) with opening/closing movements	Facial and/or jaw aching pain Limited opening Painful joint noises with opening/closing	Conservative treatment for acute cases Chronic condition may warrant multidisciplinary approach to pain management

Index

AAOS. *See* American Association of
    Orthopedic Surgeons
Abscess, 12f, 112, 112f
Absolute neutrophil count, infection risk
    and, 73t
Absolute primary polycythemia, 33
ACE inhibitors. *See* Angiotensin-converting
    enzyme inhibitors
Acetasylic acid (ASA), 53
Acid-base balance electrolyte values, 43–44
ACTH. *See* Adrenocorticotropic hormone
Actinobacillus actinomycetemcomitans, 100
Activated partial thromboplastin time
    (aPTT), 56
Addison disease, 83
ADP inhibitors, 53
Adrenal disorders, 82–88
  adrenal function tests, 83–85
  crises, 83
  insufficiency, 83
Adrenocorticotropic hormone (ACTH), 84
AFP. *See* Atypical facial pain
AHA. *See* American Heart Association
Alcohol
  bleeding risk and, 53
Aldosterone, 84
Alkaline phosphatase (ALP), 41–42
Allergic disorders, 188t
  clinical and laboratory findings, 176t–177t
  hypersensitivity reactions, 188, 188t,
    189, 190
  oral manifestations, 188–91
  patch tests, 188
  sensitization, 188
Allergic reactions, 188t
ALP. *See* Alkaline phosphatase
American Heart Association (AHA), 74
Amicar, 61
Aminocaproic acid, 61

Anemias, 33. *See also* Aplastic anemia;
    Fanconi anemia; Pernicious anemia;
    Sickle cell anemia
  classification of, 34t
  types, 34–36, 35f
Angioedema, 191
Angiotensin-converting enzyme inhibitors
    (ACE inhibitors)
  lichenoid reactions, 183
  taste changes and, 125, 125t
Angular cheilitis, 114, 115f
Antibiotic prophylaxis
  dental procedures, 73–75
  indications for, 75t
Antibiotics
  infective endocarditis, 75t
  odontogenic infections, 112, 113t
Anticoagulant drugs, 56
Antiresorptive agent, 65, 154t, 155–56
  medication-associated osteonecrosis, 12f,
    85–86, 164–67
Aplastic anemia, 38, 48f, 65
aPTT. *See* Activated partial thromboplastin time
ASA. *See* Acetasylic acid
Auscultatory gap, 29
Autoimmune conditions
  clinical and laboratory findings, 176t–177t
  oral manifestations, 171–81
  Sjögren syndrome, 171
  targeting connective tissue, 173–81
  targeting epithelium, 172–73

Bacteremia, 73
Bacterial culture. *See* Cultures
Bacterial endocarditis, 73–74
Bacterial infection
  bacterial culturing, 107, 108t–111t
  cancer treatment and, 158
  tests of, 12, 107, 112

Risk Assessment and Oral Diagnostics in Clinical Dentistry, First Edition.
Dena J. Fischer, Nathaniel S. Treister and Andres Pinto.
© 2013 John Wiley & Sons, Inc. Published 2013 by John Wiley & Sons, Inc.